TRAINING PSYCHIATRISTS FOR THE '90S:

ISSUES AND RECOMMENDATIONS

TRAINING PSYCHIATRISTS FOR THE '90S:

ISSUES AND RECOMMENDATIONS

Edited by

Carol C. Nadelson, M.D.

Carolyn B. Robinowitz, M.D.

American Psychiatric Press, Inc.

1400 K Street, N.W.
Washington, DC 20005

Manufactured in the United States of America

ISBN 0-88048-142-0

Contents

PART 3:
THE RESIDENCY PROGRAM

I. OVERVIEW

II. PROGRAM PLANNING

III. PSYCHOTHERAPY

IV. TRAINING FOR RESEARCH/TECHNOLOGY

V. SUBSPECIALIZATION

VI. EVALUATION

PART 4:
RESIDENCY PROGRAM ACCREDITATION

PART 5: FINANCING RESIDENCY TRAINING

PART 6: SUMMARY AND CONCLUSIONS

APPENDICES

Preface

The Conference, *Psychiatric Education in the 1990s*, held in Raleigh, North Carolina, April 4-5, 1986, serves as a springboard for this monograph. The authors of most of the chapters participated in the Conference, and presented thought-provoking stimulus papers. All of the participants were involved in the development of the recommendations for new directions in psychiatric education. This volume is not a compendium of Conference proceedings. It contains substantial information not presented at the Conference, and it cannot begin to impart the intense dialogue of the Conference participants, many of whose contributions are not reflected here. For that reason, we present two sets of recommendations. The concluding section of this book highlights the suggested future directions which flow from this volume. An Appendix at the end of this volume contains summaries of the discussion and recommendations of the topic-specific Conference Work Groups which grew from the stimulus papers around the Conference topics.

The editors owe a great debt of gratitude to the Steering Committee and to Conference participants, as well as to the authors of the individual chapters in this volume. Neither the Conference nor this volume would have been possible without their contribution of time, thought, and energy. We wish to thank Melvin Sabshin,

M.D., APA Medical Director, who was a constant source of ideas and support, as well as the Association for Academic Psychiatry (AAP) and the American Association of Directors of Psychiatry Residency Training (AADPRT), whose members provided counsel, leadership and expertise.

We are grateful to the organizations that supported the Conference through participation of their representatives, and who agreed to pursue and refine the Conference recommendations. Contributions from the National Institute of Mental Health and the National Institute of Alcoholism and Alcohol Abuse provided vital financial support; Institute Directors Shervert Frazier, M.D., and Robert Nivens, M.D., provided suggestions and encouragement throughout the Conference planning process. Colleagues in the private sector also provided funding and assistance: Boehringer Ingelheim Pharmaceuticals, Inc; Boots Pharaceutical, Inc.; Burroughs Wellcome Company; Charter Medical Corporation; Ciba-Geigy Corporation; DuPont Pharmaceuticals; Lederle Laboratories; Eli Lilly and Company Dista Products Company; McNeill Pharmaceutical; Mead Johnson Pharmaceutical Division; Merrell Dow Pharmaceuticals, Inc.; National Psychopharmacology Laboratories, Inc.; Pennwalt Corporation; Pfizer Inc.; Psychiatric Diagnostic Laboratories of America; Psychiatric Institutes of America; Roerig Division Pfizer, Inc.; Sandoz, Inc.; Schering Corporation; Smith, Kline and French Laboratories; E.R. Squibb and Sons, Inc.; and Upjohn Company. We especially appreciate the generosity of the Burroughs Wellcome Company which provided not only financial assistance but also support in making meeting arrangements, providing working luncheons, and hosting a banquet for participants. Clifford Parrish and Brenda Ferrell, of Burroughs Wellcome, must be singled out for their roles in Conference activities. Thanks are also due Robert O. Friedel, M.D., and Frank T. Rafferty, M.D. who contributed ideas as well as funds. The outpouring of private sector support was facilitated by the hard work of Ray Purkis, Director of APA Advertising Sales.

We would have been lost without the able assistance of Hope Z. Ball and Rosalind Keitt—respectively, Executive Secretary and Administrator of the APA Office of Education. They oversaw the arrangements and details in the planning, execution and follow-up to the Conference. We are grateful to Leslie Champlin of the APA Division of Public Affairs and Alma Herndon of Psychiatric News for developing post-conference news stories about the Conference. The production of this volume would not have been possible without the departmental support provided by Richard I. Shader, M.D., Chairman of the Department of Psychiatry of Tufts University New England Medical School and Center Hospital, and by staff members Joan Silverman, Janet Popper, and Barbara Ann Karr. APA Office of Education staff Anne M. Anders and Nora G. Phillips provided invaluable assistance during the production process. Very special gratitude is due to Teddi Fine whose editorial perseverance and creative capacities are demonstrated in the organization and fine tuning of this volume.

Carol C. Nadelson, M.D.
Carolyn B. Robinowitz, M.D.

PART 1:

PSYCHIATRIC EDUCATION IN THE '90S: AN OVERVIEW

1

INTRODUCTION:

TRAINING PSYCHIATRISTS FOR THE '90s

Carol C. Nadelson, M.D.

Carolyn B. Robinowitz, M.D.

Forces, both internal and external to psychiatry, are pressing for change in practice patterns and in residency training. Over the years, we have made many adjustments in our training programs and requirements. Today, the content, form, and structure of psychiatric residency programs must be reexamined to enable our profession to respond to the exigencies of the future.

Historically, the American Psychiatric Association has taken a leadership role in examining educational process and relating education to clinical care needs. Previous APA "decade" conferences have addressed these issues.

One of the priorities of Carol Nadelson's tenure as APA President (1985-1986) was to refocus attention on psychiatric education, in light of the substantial scientific advances in our field, as well as the prevailing economic climate. To that end, in 1985, the editors with Stefan Stein, M.D., then President of the American Association of Directors of Psychiatric Residency Training (AADPRT), to begin planning for a conference focusing on graduate education for the 1990s. A steering committee, including Alan Barnes, M.D., Jonathan Borus, M.D., Donald Fidler, M.D., Jerald Kay, M.D., Allan Tasman, M.D., and Dr. Stein, began the planning process in June 1985. The committee decided to model the conference on the very successful 1980 APA-AADPRT Conference on Manpower and Recruitment. That conference actively involved participants in developing recommendations in response to position papers or debates. These recommendations were implemented by the Conference's sponsoring organizations.

On April 4-5, 1986, the APA, in collaboration with the AADPRT, the Association of Directors of Medical Student Education in Psychiatry, and the Association for Academic Psychiatry, held a national invitational conference to recommend new directions for psychiatric education in the coming decade. The 140 attendees, experts in psychiatric education and service delivery, and representative of the major psychiatric education and service organizations, closely examined those forces which will continue to exert a major influence on the future of both psychiatric practice and the conduct of psychiatric training. These included:

- the explosive developments in science and technology, especially the neurosciences, with resulting changes in diagnosis and treatment, leading to a more sophisticated content base for education, practice, and more subspecialty/tertiary care;
- the enormous changes in health care delivery models, directed toward providing care in organized settings;
- cost containment and the "rationing" of health care;
- the rise of corporate medicine;
- the increasing need for psychiatrists in the public sector;
- the rise in the number and kind of care providers, leading to competition between and among care givers;
- the care needs of the most seriously and chronically mentally ill, as well as of those populations whose numbers are expanding, such as the elderly; and
- changing funding for and organization of academic medicine.

Conference participants addressed a host of difficult questions directly related to these changing directions in health care delivery in the U.S.:

- What are the future roles of psychiatrists? Should they increasingly serve as consultants, subspecialists, primary care givers, pharmacologists, psychotherapists? How do we and should we integrate the roles of general psychiatric practitioner and subspecialist?
- Do we have an oversupply or undersupply of psychiatrists?
- What are the emerging content areas in psychiatry in which medical students and residents should be trained?
- How should training be organized and evaluated?

- What type of faculty should assume major educational responsibility? How should faculty be utilized?
- In what settings should training occur? How should public and private sector facilities collaborate?
- Who will fund graduate medical education? What role should the government, the private sector, the patient, the student, and the profession play?
- How will we interest, recruit, and train future researchers and faculty? What career development issues are important for their retention and productivity?
- What are the ethical issues involving technology and the allocation of resources? How should they be addressed in our educational system?
- What is the impact of liability issues on psychiatric practice?

This monograph reflects the commitment of those at the conference to present theoretical concepts as well as practical recommendations for the profession. The goal of the conference and this document is to propose realistic modifications in policies and to reshape the content and format of graduate education, in order to prepare psychiatrists for practice in a changed and still changing health care environment.

2

CHALLENGES IN PSYCHIATRIC EDUCATION

Shervert H. Frazier, M.D.

Decisions about the direction of psychiatric education in the next decade will prove critical, not only to the well-being of our patients and our profession, but also to the overall quality of medical practice and health care delivery. This paper addresses questions fundamental to education and to our capacity to remain responsive to the needs of the mentally ill:

- Where will current and future psychiatric trainees practice?
- Whom will these psychiatrists treat?
- How, and through what mechanisms will future training programs be funded?
- What must be the objectives of educational programs to ensure that both psychiatrists and the delivery systems within which they practice are responsive to service needs?

Impetus to Change

Extensive change is occurring in the mental health service delivery system. Traditional hospital-based and private practice models are giving way to an increasingly wide array of alternative outpatient care models and private group practices. Practitioners must adapt to these changes, although very few have been trained to anticipate them. The wide-ranging economic and social implications of such systemic changes could not have been foreseen even as recently as a decade ago. These modifications in practice patterns necessarily will influence current and future training. Past training models do not provide young psychiatrists with needed skills and expertise to care for increasing numbers of severely ill patients seen in an expanding variety of outpatient settings. Similarly, economic considerations will have a greater impact on the locus of psychiatric training and practice. Attempts to tailor graduate education strictly to the evolving patterns and policies of reimbursement, however, could have unintended adverse effects on the nature and length of psychiatric training, as well as on the role of the psychiatrist as distinct from other mental health practitioners.

In What Settings Will Psychiatrists Practice? Whom Will They Treat?

The prevalence of major psychiatric disorders has not changed in the past two decades. Rather, the locus of care differs. Patients who were in hospitals are now in the community or on the street. Twenty years ago, we were concerned that the most severely ill persons were not receiving the best treatment possible in hospitals; we remain concerned that they are not receiving the best treatment possible outside of hospitals. We must train psychiatrists who can and are willing to treat underserved patient populations, the chronically mentally ill, minorities, the aged, and children, in both ambulatory and public sectors. While their disease process may remain relatively unchanged, the locus of their care and the biological, psychological, and social factors impinging on the nature and experience of illness may change, as a function of whether or not a patient is institutionalized. The clinical management of a patient with a psychosis in an inpatient environment differs considerably from treatment of the same patient in the community. We must prepare our students by providing training in settings and with patients they will encounter in practice. Failure to impart expertise or to foster willingness to work with the most underserved patients is tantamount to professional self-destruction. If, individually as educators and collectively as a profession, we fail to take care of the chronically and most severely mentally ill—the "lepers" of our field—we may lose the chance to care for those who have both the interest and the resources necessary to seek our care.

How Will Psychiatric Education Be Funded?

Any attempt to tailor training to clinical needs must take into account economic issues which affect practice patterns as well as training. With federal and private fiscal constraints, and in the face of specific limits on inpatient and outpatient care, how will graduate medical education be funded? The answers are not simple. The role of the federal government, particularly that of the National Institute of Mental Health (NIMH), once a major source of training funds, has changed. Since it is unlikely that the Institute will ever again have a large clinical training budget, we must think innovatively and propose boldly. Some possibilities include: a hospital "bed tax" to support training programs in settings where reimbursement is restricted; restructured pay rates for residents to enable them to pay tuition in support of their training; tax incentives to encourage corporate interests, such as the for-profit hospital sector, to underwrite the costs of education and training. We have the responsibility to work within the profession and the federal establishment to seek answers to these questions, and to propose approaches that ensure the retention and support of the goals of psychiatric education.

What Will be the Content of Psychiatric Training?

We must train psychiatrists to be physicians first, not because of any hierarchical perspective, but because they treat ill patients from a biopsychosocial frame of reference. What is called for is an "analogic" understanding of mental illness, based on and derived from an appreciation of the pathophysiology of disease as it interacts with psychological and social factors, rather than a "digital" understanding, adhering to a checklist of observable symptoms. A disadvantage of DSM-III, perhaps, is the extent to which it has adopted such a "digital" approach, permitting a variety of personnel who may have only limited understanding of and training in the broad perspectives of mental illnesses to make some diagnoses. Research advances underline this "analogic" approach. Because research is evolving rapidly, the content of psychiatric education must be sufficiently flexible to incorporate new knowledge as it emerges. Every residency program, for example, should include a mind/brain seminar, as much to stimulate intellectual excitement as to expand trainees' appreciation of the complexity of mental disorders. Intensive psychotherapeutic supervision and experience also are necessary, as is the direct teaching of interviewing skills. These lead students to develop empathy, to learn how to connect with difficult patients, and to interpret what is communicated during the interview. Our programs should emphasize a multi-faceted approach to working with the severely mentally ill, encompassing rehabilitative as well as medical skills. Moreover, students should be trained to work with colleagues within the legal and social service sectors, to ensure that requisite biopsychosocial needs are met. Further, a research experience should be a fundamental part of every psychiatrist's education. This is not a simple task. There is uneven distribution of research capacity among departments and ambivalence expressed by some educators as to the role of research in training, given the pressure for clinical and didactic experiences. This issue must be addressed and resolved because the research of today is the clinical practice of tomorrow.

Summary

Current and impending economic, personnel and service demands confronting the profession document that more than fine-tuning of the objectives of psychiatric education is needed. The convergence of several themes—the loci of psychiatric practice, the types of patients psychiatrists will attend, the need for innovation in the support of psychiatric education, the accelerating expansion of the knowledge base—all serve to underscore both the timeliness and the critical importance of the conference on psychiatric education for the '90s. The findings and recommendations contained in this monograph have significance for future decisions of NIMH and other sectors of the federal government; they are equally significant for the profession.

3

MEDICAL ACADEMICS AND ECONOMICS: CONTINUED CONFLICT OR RESOLUTION?

Carol C. Nadelson, M.D.

Carolyn B. Robinowitz, M.D.

American psychiatry faces enormous challenges for the future. The implications of the knowledge explosion in the neurosciences, psychopharmacology, and psychiatric epidemiology must be incorporated into a changing economic and political climate. While some paint a gloomy picture for the future of psychiatry, others see this as a time of great excitement and forward direction. New knowledge and innovation bring potential clinical advances, but we also must address the limits of change, responding effectively and thoughtfully in the spirit of scientific inquiry and humanism.

Medical Education: Historical Context

The history of academic medicine and medical centers in the U.S. is a relatively short one. Although the first American medical school was founded in 1765, no formal system of medical education was established until this century. Throughout the 18th and the first half of the 19th centuries, an apprenticeship model prevailed. Medical schools, which generally were proprietary institutions without academic connection, provided minimal formal didactic instruction. Physicians apprenticed themselves to those already in practice to gain clinical experience, since medical schools offered none. There was neither uniformity of the educational process nor standards for training or practice. Physicians could offer their patients little more than caring, their best judgment, and their experience. The scientific basis of modern medicine did not exist.

By the middle of the 19th century, hospitals began to develop as teaching institutions (though not yet formally connected to medical schools), and a process of selecting "house pupils" or "interns" began (1). The concept of academic medical training began to evolve during the latter part of the 19th century. Following a period of investigation, self-examination, and reconsideration, culminating in the publication of the Flexner Report in 1910 (1, 2), the change in medical education was swift and dramatic. After publication of this report, many medical schools, particularly the proprietary centers, closed, and stricter licensing requirements were instituted.

By 1920, the idea of advanced or graduate medical education had taken hold; half of all graduating physicians spent some time training and working as hospital interns. By this time, there were 15 formally recognized medical specialties. Between 1920 and 1940, accrediting bodies evolved and credentialing was instituted. Specialty boards began examining candidates for certification in the early 1930s. The development of the Office of Science Research and Development in the federal government in the early '40s led to expanded research interests and emphasized a broader concept of academic medicine, which included full-time faculty who were teachers and researchers.

By the 1960s, the focus began to shift; the era of the generalist began to give way to the era of the specialist. This change is often attributed to the emergence of a research base and the rapid expansion of knowledge and technology. Specialty training increasingly became a high priority for graduating medical students, and even larger numbers of students began to take two or more years of additional graduate training as well as formal subspecialty fellowships (3). Even the general practitioner, whose training had been as brief as a one-year rotating internship, was succeeded by the family physician—a specialist with three years of residency training, a certifying and recertifying process, and mandatory continuing medical education.

Early in its history, the cost of graduate medical education was very low, since teaching was provided primarily by volunteer faculty who donated their time. Changes in this system were fostered by a number of developments in the 1960s and early 1970s: an increasing emphasis on the involvement of academic faculty in clinical teaching as well as research, and the establishment of

Medicare in 1965 and Medicaid in 1972, which brought a unique system of access to high quality medical care. These changes in educational philosophy and reimbursement contributed to the increased demand for service and the corollary increased cost of medical education and care.

Until recently, funding for medical education came primarily from government and third-party payers. This funding was based on direct payment for teaching, on adjustments for indirect expenses, and on pass-throughs which subsidized the system, paid faculty and medical center overhead, and other costs. In addition, investigators supported by the National Institutes of Health (NIH) and the National Institute of Mental Health (NIMH) contributed greatly to medical student and resident education. These mechanisms fostered the development of complex, rigorous, high quality research, and also supported the training of a generation of physician-investigators. The era often is considered the "golden age" of medicine; it placed the United States at the forefront of medical education and research.

Greater demand for medical care also provided an impetus to increase the number of physicians practicing in the U.S. New medical schools opened, and the enrollment of foreign medical graduates (FMGs) was welcomed. Many Caribbean medical schools, not unlike the proprietary medical schools of the previous century in structure and function, were founded to accept U.S. citizens as students (1). By 1976, 20 percent of U.S. physicians were FMGs.

The tide began to turn in the late 1970s, as concern mounted that this country was overproducing physicians. This overproduction, it was reasoned, drove up the costs of medical care. By the time clearer data on the supply of physicians and the cost of medical care were available, however, many new medical schools had opened, and classes in most existing schools had doubled in size. The number of graduating medical students escalated dramatically.

Academic Medicine Today: Economics and Access

The 1980 Report of the Graduate Medical Education National Advisory Committee (GMENAC), that projected physician oversupply by the 1980s, focused on assessment of patient need and optimal care provided by physicians, not upon patient demand or supply side economics (4). At the time of its publication, neither the magnitude and cost of technologic advances nor the recent changes in patterns of health care delivery could have been predicted. Today, economists disagree on the impact of a physician oversupply. It has been estimated that each physician generates costs of $500,000 annually due to demand for and utilization of services (3). This figure has been used to suggest that decreasing the supply of physicians will lower medical care costs. At the same time, some economists predict that a physician oversupply will decrease costs because of increased competition. However, health care cannot be viewed primarily from a supply and demand perspective, nor can we naively assume that there will be no human cost in cutting the supply of physicians. Further, GMENAC addressed the non-substitutable need for physician care, not demand or cost.

Not only was it impossible in 1980 to anticipate current medical technology, but we could not have known the kinds of ethical dilemmas that would confront us as economic constraints force redefinition of medical care resources and needs. The attempt to contain medical costs by reducing the supply of physicians and services effectively rations the availability of medical care. There has been neither adequate discussion nor a rational decision-making process regarding what treatments or interventions will be rationed and how, or who will be affected by such rationing decisions. Moreover, although the concept of rationing is unpopular in the United States, it has been practiced here through the reimbursement system; current cost containment strategies will further limit access.

Unless we are willing to allocate an increasing percentage of our gross national product to health care, it is clear that we cannot continue to expend resources without regulation, and painful decision-making. For example, as currently funded, costly procedures such as organ transplants will consume an increasingly greater percentage of health care resources. We can either applaud this development and pay for it, or we can impose limits and restrictions upon its use. Whatever the choice, decisions must be explicit. Thurow has pointed out that "health care costs do not represent a problem simply of economics or rampant technology, but a problem of ethics and social priorities" (6).

In addition to its potential impact on patient care, a major consequence of cost containment is the reduction of funding for research and training; this can alter the future for generations to come. It implies accepting limits on our productivity and on the development of new information and technology. The difficult trade-offs brought by economic constraints are particularly problematic for Americans who are used to "having it all." The focus on cost and cost containment, contrasted to optimal care and patient need, will force us to look at priorities and consider the types of sacrifice we are willing to make.

Changing Economics of Care: Changing Economics of Education

The complex interaction among education, economics and patient care must be addressed. The growth of the academic medical center and its current crisis must be understood. By 1985, there were 5,000 residency programs and 23 specialty boards in the U.S. (3). Although residency training occurs in 1,700 hospitals, 46 percent of all residents have been trained in just 100 teaching hospitals (5). Thus, the academic medical center has become the major site for post-graduate training in the U.S.

The financing of medical education has continued to be based on cross-subsidization, depending primarily on patient care revenues and charges, with increasing costs being borne not by patients themselves, but by third-party payers, or even "fourth-" party payers (employers). For hospitals, the losses incurred by caring for the poor have continued to be shared between public and private sectors. Currently, between 81 and 87 percent of graduate medical education is financed through patient revenues (5). While the cost of graduate medical education represents only 2 percent of total health care expenditures, the latter has been estimated to be $400 billion per year; thus the expense of graduate medical education is substantial (5). Clearly, then, proposed and emerging changes in reimbursement systems will generate fiscal problems for academic centers, with enormous implications for both training and education.

Teaching hospitals are reported to have substantially higher operating costs per discharged Medicare patient than non-teaching hospitals; 126 percent greater, by one estimate (5). When this figure is factored and analyzed, it appears that 19 percent of the cost is related to case mix (teaching hospitals tend to have sicker patients, even with the same diagnosis), 14 percent to differences in area wage levels (teaching hospitals are more likely to be in urban, high wage areas), 18 percent to numbers of beds in the facility (more beds are more costly, and teaching hospitals have more beds), 12 percent to the location of the hospitals (there are higher costs and proportionally poorer patients in urban areas; costs are as much as 70 percent higher in population centers of over 2 million people), and about 14 percent related to the indirect costs of medical education (including ancillary services, extra tests, procedures, and additional time spent by personnel because of the educational mission of the institution) (3). Any or all of these factors can be addressed separately or together; they are not, however, unrelated.

Another expensive component of the educational process often not considered in discussions of educational costs, is the cost of the credentialing and accreditation processes. The mechanisms that implement the evaluation of performance are elaborate and expensive, but they also enhance quality assurance. Proposals to expand the variety of care delivery systems and levels of care provided will necessitate the development of new evaluative and accrediting measures, and require substantial revision of training programs. Thus, if health care personnel are to continue to deliver high quality care, costs are likely to increase, at least temporarily.

Still another factor adding to the costs of the current health care system is the increase in numbers of specialists who have been trained in the last few decades. These physicians often practice in communities close to the sites at which they trained, and tend to provide complex, tertiary care. It has been suggested that much of this tertiary care represents an "oversupply." Similarly, those highly trained specialists and subspecialists who provide primary care because there are not enough patients with subspecialty needs, have been regarded as "overtrained" and too expensive!

These specialists often turn community hospitals into tertiary care facilities which then compete with academic medical centers for patients. While such settings may give rise to escalating costs and duplicative services, they also deliver high quality care, readily accessible to large numbers of patients. Since limitations have not been placed on either the number of physicians in specialties or subspecialties, or on the locations of their practice, supply appears to have increased, rather than decreased demand.

Many communities are reported to have large numbers of empty hospital beds which are expensive to maintain. In some areas, academic medical centers have been able to save money by affiliating with community hospitals to provide a network of care delivery and to eliminate duplicative services across facilities. This approach requires a spirit of cooperation; but sharing resources is not fostered by an excessive emphasis on the procompetitive model.

Yet another dimension of the problem of funding health care delivery is the administrative costs of the bureaucracy that has grown up around the structure and organization of the delivery system (7). "Administrative waste" is cited as a reason for escalating costs in the U.S. In Great Britain and Canada administrative costs are lower. The potential savings, if administrative costs were contained, could provide more funds for patient care.

Economics and Research

The pressure for academic medical centers to be fiscally viable will affect the educational process in complex ways. In addition to providing reimbursement for education (including salaries, facilities, etc), the funding mechanisms established during the last several decades also enabled salaried physicians to direct some of their attention to research, as well as to their clinical and educational activities. As noted, research grants have provided academic medical centers an important educational support base. Taken together, a complex system of cross-subsidies and earnings has produced unprecedented and truly extraordinary investigative and educational enterprises.

The future of academic medicine and research also depends upon the training of the next generation of investigators; academic medical centers have been the model for such activity. It is not enough for medical schools to train new practitioners. These schools must be models for inquiry and life-long continuing education, as Flexner indicated 75 years ago.

Special Educational Dilemmas

In addition to the broader conceptual, economic, and ethical issues we have considered, specific educational problems are raised by the altered patterns of the health care delivery system. Changes in the distribution and means of providing services, and in reimbursement mechanisms imply corresponding fundamental change in educational structure and organization. For example, what is the impact on the learning experience of students and residents who care primarily for patients with very short-term hospital stays, who are part of an ambulatory health maintenance network? Clearly, there will be less time to care for hospitalized patients, and the focus will be on those in acute distress. Many surgical patients, for example, will receive their pre-operative workups in ambulatory settings with evaluation provided by one resident; the patients then will enter the hospital the morning of surgery where another resident will take responsibility for peri-operative care; follow-up will be provided by yet another resident. There will not be much time for residents to learn about long-term or chronic illnesses, or to follow patients in multiple care settings. The same type of fragmentation of care is likely to occur with psychiatric patients.

Paradoxically, since chronic illness is more likely to be the focus of future health care needs, as our population ages, there will be a greater need for clinicians experienced in long term care and chronic illness. Trainees will have difficulty following these patients in a system that fractionates care, facilities, and providers. The structure of our current medical education system will not fulfill the learning needs of future physicians.

Medical consultation provides another example of the complexity of the problems engendered by the changing health care system. Its availability and use have always been a major component of medical education and clinical training. The process of learning from more experienced colleagues, sometimes in other disciplines and specialties, not only has direct benefits for the patient, but also is a model for the physician's future learning, providing impetus for the lifelong acquisition of new skills, information and knowledge. Unfortunately, there is now a built-in disincentive to utilizing consultation either for patient or physician benefit. Scientific growth and clinical trials may be substantially reduced because the payment system minimizes use of additional services, especially consultation, and the use or consideration of new technology.

The current, and most likely future, health care delivery system rewards hospitals for treating patients at lower costs. It encourages care givers (through hospital-generated or related pressures) to order less costly care (tests and procedures) for their patients, and to discharge or transfer them earlier in the course of treatment. Reimbursement levels for care may become a ceiling rather than a floor, further threatening to compromise the quality of care.

Our current reimbursement structure also rewards organizations that provide ambulatory care or that emphasize minimal service system use. Treatment decisions may be made less on the basis of patient need or severity of illness, and more on financial considerations. Little decision-making is based upon either educational or research objectives. The "teaching patient" of the '50s and '60s is gone!

Although brief ambulatory treatment, whether in an HMO or other setting, will utilize fewer resources and may be beneficial to some patients, the pressure for haste may limit careful diagnostic assessment. When a patient is hospitalized, there may be covert pressure to consider, even to choose, a diagnosis that would permit a longer length of stay.[1] This approach could undermine the gains

---

[1]The Prospective Payment System, created for the Medicare program as part of the Social Security Amendments of 1983, established a series of 168 so-called Diagnosis Related Groupings (DRGs). These DRGs set maximum lengths of stay and corollary prospective payments based upon diagnosis. Through this payment mechanism, which

in applying rational science to diagnosis that are embodied in DSM-III and damage emerging epidemiologic efforts. In addition, discharge-transfer-readmission tactics may be used to reduce the lengths of stay, leading to premature patient discharge. Further, psychological testing or additional laboratory tests may be performed less frequently because of their cost to the system. Again, the implications for trainees are obvious.

There also may be limitations in the types of treatment that will be used. For example, psychopharmacologic treatment of major affective disorders requires some time for its impact to be determined. Teaching hospitals and psychiatrists caring for these patients will be under pressure to discharge patients rapidly. Thus, a suicidally depressed patient may be treated with electroconvulsive therapy (ECT) to avoid the potential delay in response to the use of tricyclics. Although the choice of ECT as a treatment modality may be appropriate and beneficial for some patients, treatment determinations may be modified by anticipated time of response, an issue that should be but one of many factors influencing therapeutic choice. Trainees, then, may not learn to make treatment decisions based primarily on clinical indications. Pressures to make cost effective treatment decisions may increase physician concern about liability issues. Physicians, increasingly under pressure to "treat the chart" and not the patient, working out of fear, not just clinical judgment, could be pulled in opposing directions simultaneously. On the one hand, they will be required to limit investigation to "necessary" testing to be more "cost effective"; on the other hand, they will feel increased pressure to practice "defensive psychiatry" because of libility concerns. Trainees, thus, may learn little about either the use or cost of tests or the setting of clinical priorities.

The Future of the Teaching Hospital

The teaching hospital may become a "last resort" hospital, used only, or primarily, for those patients requiring the most complex

---

may serve as a model for third-party reimbursement, facilities are paid a fixed sum, based on diagnosis, without regard to a patient's length of stay (LOS). If the LOS is shorter than the DRG, the facility gains income over expenses; if the LOS is longer, the facility incurs the added cost. Thus, facilities may try to select diagnoses with longer LOS to enhance profits, and to "cover" themselves for longer LOS.

tertiary care facilities. Accordingly, "routine" patients may seek treatment in lower cost community hospitals, or may choose private, unaffiliated facilities with more luxurious quarters and better marketing. Such a future course not only would have a negative impact upon costs of teaching hospitals, but also would alter the patient population seen there. Trainees would then observe fewer routine illnesses, and be more apt to treat more severely ill and less affluent patients. The atypical or nonresponding patient could become the norm, particularly on a referral basis.

The other side of the coin is the search for "simple" patients and the corollary, avoidance of more complex patients. Thus, patients with personality disorders with multiple hospitalizations, or patients with atypical or unresponsive depressions, may be referred away from the very settings that could provide the most assistance. Trainees may be denied these learning opportunities as well.

Trainees will be exposed less frequently to the natural history of illness or rehabilitation; long-term treatment may be relegated to special, usually public institutions, further limiting residents' exposure to chronic and more severe illness. Moreover, we are already beginning to see evidence that as lengths of stay are shortened, the intensity of care and number of admission workups will increase, leading to overwork (or over-experience in certain areas) of house staff. There will be increasing need for additional house staff, nonphysicians, or non-trainee physicians to provide services. These other providers may support a two-class system of performance and care.

Psychiatry: The Future

For psychiatry, some of the changes in the health care delivery system may have even more serious implications than for other specialties. Information about psychiatric illness continues to be shrouded in myth, mystery and pessimism. Financial cutbacks may seriously affect research and education, limiting the potential for continued scientific advances and information dissemination. The stigma of mental illness today is much like the stigma of many other illnesses, such as tuberculosis, a century ago. Will mental illness receive even less attention in the future than it has in recent years?

Among the advances on the horizon are maps of specificity for neurotransmitters and receptors, an expanding understanding of the mechanisms of action of pharmacological agents, brain imaging techniques, emerging epidemiologic data, elucidation of genetic patterns for major mental disorders, increased understanding of mechanisms and treatment for diseases such as Alzheimer's, the ability through longitudinal studies to identify at-risk populations early in life, innovative behavioral and psychological interventions, greater understanding of mind-brain interrelationships, productive psychotherapeutic efficacy studies, delineation of mechanisms and treatments of substance abuse, and understanding of the contributions of psychological and life experience factors to physical illness.

New psychiatric problems continue to appear as old ones resurface. For example, the neuropsychiatric implications of AIDS have recently emerged as a major unforeseen problem. At the same time, we see an escalation of problems such as family violence and substance abuse. If our projections are short-term or based on past experience alone, it is not always possible to anticipate new developments and to account for them in our planning. We must continue to explore new avenues and not trade off one disorder for another. Had not an investment been made to advance our knowledge of basic immunology, biochemistry, and epidemiology, recent advances in our understanding of AIDS could never have occurred. In many ways, current arguments favoring nonacademic and proprietary settings for training mirror those of a century ago. However, the values and rigor of the current process have produced unprecedented advances. At times, it seems that we have almost forgotten the enormous progress made in a very short time and the danger we face if we precipitously change course.

Consideration must be given to developing funding systems that reward preventive approaches, but do not punish development or use of technology. Such interventions, although initially costly, may eventually decrease the overall cost of patient care. We must be clear about our priorities and refrain from being caught up in the rhetoric of economics or the politics of systems.

References

1. Ludmerer K: Learning to Heal. New York, Basic Books, 1985
2. Flexner A: Medical Education in the United States and Canada: A Report to the Carnegie Foundation for the Advancement of Teaching. New York, The Carnegie Foundation, 1910

3. Preliminary Report of the New York State Commission on Graduate Medical Education. New York, September, 1985
4. Office of Graduate Medical Education, Health Resources Administration: Report of the Graduate Medical Education National Advisory Committee. Washington DC, Department of Health and Human Services publication #HRA 81-652, 1980
5. Task Force on Academic Health Centers: Prescription for Change—Report of the Task Force on Academic Health Centers. New York, The Commonwealth Fund, 1985
6. Thurow L: Learning to say no. NEJM 311:1569-1572, 1984
7. Himmelstein DU, Woolhandler S: Cost without benefit: Administrative waste in U. S. health care. NEJM 314:441-445, 1986

4

ACADEMIC CAREERS IN PSYCHIATRY: FACULTY DEVELOPMENT AND RETENTION

Norbert B. Enzer, M.D.

The boundaries of academic psychiatry are very broad; within it are found psychiatrists with diverse theoretical orientation and interests, working in every conceivable setting. Although academic psychiatry is not the sole provider of psychiatric education, it does have a special responsibility for, and it exerts a powerful influence on education and, therefore, on the future practice of psychiatry. It also has a responsibility for the development of new understanding and knowledge, and for more effective approaches to the assessment and treatment of patients. Less attention, however, has been directed to the comprehensive development of academic psychiatrists than to development in other areas of psychiatric practice.

Until quite recently, support for academic medicine, including academic psychiatry, seemed almost unlimited. Opportunities for those interested in academic careers were everywhere. From 1948, when the National Institute of Mental Health (NIMH) was created, until quite recently, clinical training and education had been a high priority for the federal government. Support was available for both faculty and resident stipends in general and child psychiatry. Individuals who wished to pursue academic teaching careers were supported by NIMH Career Teacher Awards. These programs did much to increase the numbers of psychiatrists and were influential in establishing and strengthening American medical school departments of psychiatry and improving psychiatric education.

Times have changed, and American medicine, including medical education, is undergoing changes of a magnitude not previously experienced. The rapid expansion of knowledge and technology, changes in the demographic character of the population, alterations in the patterns of disease and in the need for health and mental health care, new developments in the organization of medical practice and care delivery, professional education, and research require concomitant change in the institutions responsible for the development of future generations of psychiatrists.

The organization, settings, and content of psychiatric education will be modified. Difficult decisions will be required, and they will need to be made wisely. New knowledge, and perhaps new categories of patients and clinical experiences will have to be accommodated, while preserving certain of the traditions and perspectives of the past. Whatever else is involved, psychiatric education depends fundamentally on three groups of people: those who wish to enter the profession, patients with whom trainees may interact, and faculty willing to teach, serve as models, and think hard and clearly about what should be provided.

A number of questions must be considered. How many faculty members should there be in academic departments of psychiatry? How many of these people should be psychiatrists? How should they be supported? What should their qualifications be? What should they do? This paper will focus on these questions as they relate to psychiatrist faculty employed by academic institutions. Questions of recruitment and retention of new academic psychiatrists also will be addressed.

Education and Adademic Psychiatry: Historical Perspective

In the last twenty years, academic psychiatry attracted individuals whose interests ranged across a variety of fields: human development, normal psychological and social functioning, psychosocial concomitants of medical illness, the effects of psychological and social events on the body's functions, patient interviewing and doctor-patient relationships, and other topics. In part because of past support for psychiatric education by the NIMH, many psychiatrists with interest in teaching found opportunities in academic departments of psychiatry.

Psychiatry has taken its educational responsibilities seriously, devoting substantial effort to define its educational mission, refine its programs and develop its educators. The NIMH Career Teacher Awards of the 1950s and 1960s produced a number of psychiatrists who continue to have substantial influence on psychiatric education. Unfortunately, notwithstanding efforts to strengthen the cadre of academic psychiatrists, leaders in this field remain a minority in the profession.

The report of the 1975 Lake of the Ozarks conference on psychiatric education, *Psychiatric Education: Prologue to the 1980s*, stated: "Despite great stress on the importance of good psychiatric teaching and the widespread participation of psychiatrists as teachers (some 63 percent of all psychiatrists do some teaching), there seems to be relatively little systematic attention given to the formal development of teaching skill in psychiatrists" (1). That statement may be as true today as it was then.

Clinical education in medicine has depended upon the willingness of clinicians to teach and supervise medical students and residents, and to serve as role models. For most of the history of American medicine, those clinician-educators have been practicing physicians, taking students and residents "under their wings" and doing so largely on a voluntary basis. Only in the last half of this century has American medical education seen a significant growth in the numbers of full-time faculty in the clinical disciplines; the growth of clinical departments in medical schools since the end of World War II has been nothing short of phenomenal. Along with these developments, new medical schools were established, their class sizes increased, and the number, size, and diversity of programs of graduate medical education expanded.

With this growth, psychiatry, as other specialties, has also continued to rely on those engaged primarily in clinical practice to serve as educators. The Lake of the Ozarks Conference report noted that "There is extensive division of labor among faculty members, with "full time" faculty members bearing...the greatest administrative responsibility for residency program form and content, but part-time and voluntary faculty members carrying great responsibility for day-to-day didactic and clinical education of residents" (1).

As noted in the previous chapter by Nadelson and Robinowitz, earlier in this century, training was largely the responsibility of hospitals, not medical schools. More recently, academic departments have assumed greater responsibilities for graduate medical education, and there is continuing pressure to do so. For that reason, teaching skills alone are not sufficient. The educator must be knowledgeable about program planning, educational strategies and techniques, and the assessment of program effectiveness and student evaluation. This knowledge is particularly vital as leadership, standards, and quality control of graduate education have become the responsibility of academic departments of psychiatry.

It is uncertain whether we will be able to rely on the continued good will and contributed time of practitioner-teachers. However, while academic departments should assume more responsibility for direct teaching, they also should provide teaching-practitioners the opportunity to refine their skills as dictated by changes in educational strategy and program direction.

Roles and Functions of Faculty

The academic institutions in which contemporary graduate education in psychiatry occurs, must work increasingly with external agencies, insurance companies, employers, professional organizations, accrediting bodies, labor unions, the courts, voluntary citizens groups and others. Even university medical centers which, in the past, enjoyed special autonomy, are now caught up in the requirements for accountability, procedures to assure fairness and equal opportunity, measures of quality assurance, and mechanisms of cost containment. The functions of faculty within the constraints of these administrative and procedural complexities are equally diverse.

Academic Psychiatrists as Educators

Residency programs in psychiatry incorporate training and education. Training implies the development, through instruction and drill, of certain skills. Professional education implies the acquisition of a body of knowledge, and it incorporates values, traditions, attitudes, and styles. Residency programs, thus, must instill an appreciation of history, a literacy in the field, an analytic approach to problem solving, a capacity to evaluate new knowledge and technology, and a thorough knowledge of the principal focus of the discipline. Residency program graduates must be able to think about what they do, continually considering the possibilities of improved or more effective solutions within a circumscribed ethical standard. At the same time, they must be master technologists, able to apply their knowledge and skills with wisdom and compassion.

It is the faculty that creates the human environment in which a program of psychiatric education is embedded. That environment should be one of inquiry, scholarship, excitement, and quality patient care. The Report of the Lake of the Ozarks Conference suggested a series of psychiatric faculty responsibilities which articulate the educational function:

1. serving as role models, demonstrating, through their own example, how a mature clinician should approach the diagnosis and care of patients;
2. supervising and guiding residents as they develop their own skills by providing advice, support, information, and extensive evaluative feedback;
3. conveying essential information concerning the intellectual and theoretical foundation of psychiatry through both clinical and didactic teaching;
4. serving as sensors to the developments in the immediate and larger social milieu, the profession, and the relevant sciences; communicating these to residents; and shaping the educational program to keep pace not only with the present but the future;
5. continually expanding their own state of knowledge and skill so that what is preached is practiced as well;
6. acting as compassionate, perceptive guides to professional development (with special skills honed by professional training) who can be responsive to the individual needs of residents at a time of great stress and growth;[1]
7. understanding and respecting residents sufficiently to include them in major decisions that affect their education and professional well-being and shaping the residency program, to the extent possible to achieve a reasonable balance between the fulfillment of resident needs, professional responsibility, and the demands of the service setting;
8. serving as the legally and professionally responsible representative of patients' best interests and exerting leadership to assure that residents, as well as faculty members, practice with those interests foremost;
9. participating in administrative decisions that affect the educational milieu; the curriculum; faculty; residents and other students in the training settings; the use of time, space, and personnel; the dominant philosophy and approaches to education; and the accommodation among departmental research, education, and service activities;
10. helping to articulate educational objectives, assessing whether and how well they are being met by teachers and students, and

---

[1] While this role should not be confused with that of therapist, at times, faculty members may be called on to exercise their diagnostic skill and refer some residents to appropriate professional help when needed.

introducing those changes that are needed to aid in their realization (1).

Academic Psychiatrists: The Other Key Roles

The foregoing list defines the responsibilities of academic faculty principally in terms of the residency program. As we know, very few faculty are devoted solely to teaching residents. The collective roles and functions of the faculty of an academic department of psychiatry extend far beyond educational activities:

- They serve as leaders, decision-makers, and administrators within the department, the medical school, the hospital, and other clinical settings with regard to policy formation, planning, and implementation in education, research, patient care, public service, personnel, space and resource allocation, and finances.
- They serve as advocates for the discipline, promoting by example, proclamation, and documentation of the field of psychiatry.
- They serve as advocates for the mentally ill.
- They provide expert assistance to sources of funding for psychiatric care, research and education, and to those planning future developments.
- They provide information and expert opinion to legislative and governmental executive bodies and various social agencies regarding the needs for psychiatric care and developments in the field.
- They instruct medical students, residents in psychiatry and other specialties, and sometimes students in allied health and mental health disciplines. The teaching activities include individual supervision, seminars, case conferences, ward rounds, lectures, and many other instructional formats. The content includes the interactional skills, the assessment of clinical data, the formulation of a biopsychosocial understanding of patients, diagnosis, skills in consultation, knowledge of psychopathology and the various approaches to psychiatric treatment, and many other topics.
- They evaluate the progress of individual students and residents, develop assessment procedures, write examination questions, set standards and participate in promotional decisions.
- They advise students and residents of their educational programs and the problems they may encounter, the selection of elective experiences, their future training and career direction.
- They occasionally may perform psychiatric evaluation of students, faculty, and staff for administrative purposes.
- They develop instructional materials.

- They develop and monitor the curriculum and participate with others in the approval of curricula for various students.
- They participate in the selection and admission of medical students and residents; they serve on search and selection committees for new faculty, and on promotions committees.
- They do research, write and make scholarly presentations.
- They provide direct patient care and administer clinical services.
- They provide administrative supervision of the clinical work of residents.
- They participate in program evaluation regarding education and clinical activities.
- They prepare written proposals for external financial support of research, educational programs, clinical services, and demonstration programs; and manage grant funds when received.
- They participate in the preparation of applications and reports for accreditation review of educational and clinical service programs.
- They plan and participate in programs of continuing medical education, continuing their own professional development; they are involved in the activities of professional organizations.
- They serve as reviewers and critics of the work of other; and provide formal and informal consultants to other physicians, educators, and researchers.
- They participate in activities relevant to quality assurance, risk management, and cost containment.
- They assist in the development of new and younger faculty.

Although the list includes some activities which may apply to many faculty members, it also includes some which apply to only a few. The particular activities of any one faculty member would likely include a number of these specific tasks. The relative importance of a single activity depends on a number of factors, some of which may be idiosyncratic to a particular institution or person.

Despite the fact that most institutions proclaim their primary commitment to be to education, evidence of scholarship—research and publications—is the single most important factor upon which promotion and tenure decisions are made. Excellence in teaching alone may be recognized at best by a plaque or certificate; even educational leadership, unless accompanied by published evidence of scholarship, is not likely to lead to academic advancement. Although there are variations among institutions regarding the standards and the "toughness" of the process of advancement, there does seem to be a general trend toward research oriented standards.

Thus, there is great variation in the roles played by academic psychiatrists, and little reward for many of their activities, making both recruitment and retention of these professionals all the more difficult.

Recruitment and Maintenance of Faculty

In psychiatry, there has been a relatively constant flow of young people interested in academic careers, and, until recently, there have been abundant opportunities. Beginning in the early 1970s, the availability of external support for psychiatric education decreased. As competition for research support has increased, university funding of departments of psychiatry has slowed, and in some cases, declined. At the time that departments of psychiatry and other institutions with residency programs became more dependent upon funds generated through clinical services, the pressures for cost containment and of competition for available clinical service dollars have increased.

Individual career decisions by medical students and young physicians have been influenced by these and other economic and social changes. The burden of debt experienced by students at the end of medical school adds a new factor which must be considered in both career choice and decisions about post-graduate training. The opportunities, constraints, and limitations of a career in academic psychiatry must be taken into account by students and residents. How these various institutional and personal factors will affect future recruitment in academic psychiatry is unclear, but it is safe to assume that they will not have a positive impact.

Like all other "futures" discussions, those relating to the coming generation of academic psychiatrists and psychiatric educators are fraught with uncertainties. Among other things, there is a need to know a great deal more about faculty members and about the departments of psychiatry in which they work. We need to know more about the characteristics, professional history and activities of successful academic psychiatrists, and about the nature, composition and organization of good departments. We need to know how a faculty divides its collective time, how it assigns tasks and responsibilities, and how its members are compensated.

Three related and overlapping areas must be addressed as we consider future faculty development. First, there is a need to create and nurture an interest in academic psychiatry among residents, medical students, and perhaps even among pre-medical students. They need to see the field as intellectually interesting and challenging, and they need to be informed about opportunities, requirements and limitations. Second, there is a need to provide preparation for an academic career and for continuing career development. These two areas of concern are directly related to recruitment. The third area is concerned with the retention of psychiatrists in academia.

Recruitment: Developing an Interest

The developments in the past thirty-five years, a period which incorporates the entire lifetimes of most psychiatric residents and medical students, illustrates the pace of change in psychiatry. Discussion of successes as well as failures and dead-end paths that have been pursued would help develop an awareness of the necessary skills and the tolerance of frustration needed to pursue a career in academic psychiatry. Certainly, some of these perspectives could be included in course work and clinical experiences to which medical students and residents are exposed; some might be provided through electives or extracurricular activities.

Students and residents in psychiatry need to have direct contact with investigators and scholars working in the field. Unfortunately, the very people who might be most stimulating to medical students and residents with potential for academic careers, are often inaccessible. Means must be found to provide exposure to successful academicians and investigators. Research seminars should be open to medical students and residents. Faculty members need to be encouraged to participate in medical school elective research programs.

Departments of psychiatry need to make it their business to seek out students who may have academic interests. Admission offices and student affairs staff can be helpful in this process; psychiatry clubs or voluntary discussion groups may attract others. Those students and residents who can be identified as interested and who seem to have the intellectual and personal characteristics of academic psychiatrists, must be the focus of particular and deliberate attention.

Career Development

Those wishing to pursue academic careers will need training beyond residency. Research fellowships or advanced training with exposure to clinical research are a requisite for faculty appointments in other areas of medicine. As yet, this is not the case in academic psychiatry, although the profession is moving in that direction. Questions arise about how such additional training can be arranged and supported, and whether those interested can afford to continue training in view of their debts and the uncertainty of academic appointments.

In the past, a variety of mechanisms, more readily available to individuals and institutions, allowed some individuals to take advantage of post-residency training. Unfortunately, many of those support mechanisms no longer exist or are so limited as to be truly discouraging. Even with an increase in the number of post-residency programs, they will not be available in all departments, requiring many interested graduates to make geographic moves.

Some institutions might develop formal "academic tracks" within their residency programs, recognizing that support for the additional time would have to be provided. With careful planning and appropriate advice, medical students with interest in and potential for academic careers might be counseled to seek initial residency appointments at institutions that provide such special tracks or advanced post-residency training.

Formal preparation for an academic psychiatry career, whether during residency or in post-residency fellowship, blends with the less formal processes of faculty development. In general, the need for opportunities to continue to develop skills and knowledge, support and encouragement in that effort, and to feel appreciated and valued are essential. Time and willing assistance of senior colleagues are the most important elements.

In the past, "survival of the fittest" was often the predominant approach to faculty development. Individual tenacity, and aggressiveness largely determined the outcome. Although some may have received guidance, protection, and assistance, more often the aid provided was serendipitous. With the changes occurring in psychiatry, including the increasing financial burdens of the training years, the field may be unwise to rely on the patterns of the past. Reliance upon past practices may be institutionally wasteful and imprudent, as well as personally unkind and unfair.

As the new economics of health care and medical education are increasingly felt by academic medical centers, departments of psychiatry will have to work harder and more deliberately to maintain the kind of environment in which scholarship, research, and high quality education can flourish. Faculty interest in developing new understanding, the challenge of the unknown, the fascination with knowledge, its structure and organization, and the means by which it is transferred to others, needs to be nurtured and protected. Young academicians need interactions with colleagues—interactions which take time, and against which other responsibilities must be balanced.

A fine balance must be struck between the opportunity to do something at the right time and excessive protection, between responsibilities assigned too soon and opportunities offered too late. There is a risk of exploitation, of assignments from which little is learned, little satisfaction is derived, and for which little credit is given.

There is also a need for more formal instruction in research methods, teaching strategies and techniques, grant application preparation, or administrative procedures. Some of this teaching may be approached on an individual tutorial basis or in workshops or seminars.

Faculty Retention

Although the retention of young faculty is inextricably linked to career development, a few specific issues must be addressed. Faculty must feel valued, and they must have a level of personal and professional satisfaction which permits them to persist in their academic careers. They must be adequately compensated, and in a manner that permits pursuit of academic activities, rather than income generating activities. The reliance upon faculty for income generation is a problem that is likely to intensify. Economic competition for bright young people will continue, and those young faculty members who may be overburdened by activities only tangentially related to the academic environment may choose to leave it.

Some institutions have responded to the competing needs for income generation and scholarly pursuits by creating a two-track system in which two groups of full-time faculty exist side by side. One group provides patient care, generates income, and provides the bulk of medical student and resident clinical instruction. The other group cares only for a limited number of patients (often related to clinical research activities), generates research income through grants, conducts research, and provides for research training. The latter group often enjoys the benefits of tenure, sabbatical leaves and other ammenities of regular faculty appointment. The former may have a somewhat higher income level.

Reward systems, particularly academic advancement, need to be modified to place less emphasis on research success and publication. Many of the other functions of faculty are essential to the maintenance of a department of psychiatry. A few faculty are truly distinguished teachers who approach their work in a particularly scholarly fashion. They may imbue their students with a sense of inquiry through their capacity to synthesize information and to create new hypotheses even though they are not active investigators. It seems a shame that a credible method of assessing excellence and scholarship other than through publication lists has not been found.

Conclusion

Career development in academic psychiatry must become a higher priority, requiring time, resources, and thought. Much of the responsibility inevitably will rest with departments of psychiatry and with the academic health centers. Chairpersons must make it clear that academic psychiatry career development is a high priority, and make it possible for the necessary time and resources to be available. However, the responsibilities extend beyond the chairperson to each member of the faculty. The intellectual and personal environment of a department of psychiatry is determined by the people who work within it. If a department is to attract and retain young people who can contribute, it must welcome and support them.

The field of psychiatry itself has some responsibility as well. It is the academic enterprise which will supply the practitioners and knowledge of the future. As a result, all of psychiatry should have a vested interest in assuring that there is an adequate supply of new faculty, and that the academic departments of psychiatry continue to be exciting places in which to work and to train.

Reference

1. Rosenfeld AH: Psychiatric Education: Prologue to the 1980s: Report of the Conference on Education in Psychiatry, Lake of the Ozarks, Missouri. Washington, DC, American Psychiatric Association, 1976

PART 2:

SELECTION AND ADMISSION OF TRAINEES

Despite the problems in the application and acceptance processes for psychiatric residency training, increasing numbers of talented medical students are entering our profession. Kay presents an overview of the gains made by the specialty in the six years since the 1980 conference on psychiatric recruitment and manpower. He indicates that as the specialty faces new challenges to its future in the form of diminished support for psychiatric training, and new economic factors influencing the shape and content of future practice, these gains may not continue. We must reexamine and correct problems inherent in our recruitment and selection processes, if we are to move into the next decade strong in the number and quality of new psychiatrists.

In his second article, Kay discusses the criteria for and the process of selection of psychiatric residents. He suggests that the positive changes made in the Special Requirements (Essentials) governing residencies must be augmented by the establishment of new, formal admission criteria by our residency training programs.

Stein underscores the need for increased attention by psychiatric educators to the transition from medical school to residency, beginning with the application process. He analyzes the complex, often haphazard manner in which the National Residency Matching Program (NRMP) occurs, a Match in which not all prospective resi-

dents and training programs participate. He suggests a host of mechanisms to achieve greater precision, responsibility, and satisfaction in the matching process.

The overarching question of the adequacy of the supply of psychiatrists to meet future needs also is dissected. If we correct our recruitment and selection problems, becoming even more stringent in our admission criteria, will we fail to meet the demands for psychiatric services in the 1990s? Alternatively, will the new rigor draw increasing numbers to our specialty, moving from the past shortage to excess?

Jerald Kay, M.D.
Stefan Stein, M.D.

5

FOLLOW-UP OF THE 1980 RECRUITMENT CONFERENCE

Jerald Kay, M.D.

In 1980, after nearly a decade during which a diminishing percentage of medical students entered psychiatry, a national conference on psychiatric manpower and recruitment was convened. Data collected by the American Psychiatric Association (APA), the American Medical Association (AMA), the Association of American Medical Colleges (AAMC), and the National Resident Matching Program (NRMP) had indicated a constant decline in the percent of American students who were choosing psychiatry as a specialty. In 1968, psychiatrists represented 12 percent of all residents. By 1980, only 2.7 percent of U.S. seniors entered a PGY-1 in psychiatry. Ironically, this decline was occurring at the same time that the Graduate Medical Education National Advisory Committee (GMENAC) projected a serious shortage of psychiatrists.

The 1980 conference examined the reasons for recruitment problems, and focused on a number of specific areas of concern: (1) the process of medical student admission and selection; (2) the character and content of medical education and the socialization of students; (3) psychiatry's image; (4) careers in psychiatry; (5) the relationship between psychiatry and primary care medicine; and (6) the psychiatric residency training program.

Specific strategies were developed for improved recruitment. These were implemented by a number of educational organizations. The conference's key considerations and recommendations included:

1. Psychiatry should heighten its visibility during the college years, since experiences at this time often determine whether a student will choose medicine and then psychiatry, or clinical psychology. Psychiatry is not well understood by undergraduates. It is rarely discussed outside the context of the pre-med program, and pre-med advisors have only a limited understanding of the specialty. Since psychology has a substantially higher profile in the undergraduate years, psychiatrists should participate in pre-med clubs, work with pre-med advisors, and involve themselves in student health services if the field is to attract more students.
2. Medical student teaching should be a high priority for departments of psychiatry.
3. The federal government could improve recruitment into the field by reinstating the Career Teacher program and increasing the number of medical student stipends.
4. Junior faculty should be rewarded for teaching accomplishments as well as for research.
5. Introductory medical school behavioral science courses, providing important initial student contact with psychiatry, should be taught by enthusiastic, motivated psychiatrist-clinicians.
6. The development of psychiatry clubs should be encouraged as effective means of promoting relationships among students and faculty, and nurturing student interest in the field.
7. Student clerkships providing experience in acute patient care should be developed to demonstrate the efficacy of psychiatric intervention, reinforcing a positive image of the specialty.
8. The academic rigor of psychiatric courses should be comparable to that of courses in other departments.
9. Research should be undertaken to ascertain how and when students make choices to enter medicine and to specialize in a particular discipline.
10. Active, unambivalent student recruitment is both effective and necessary.
11. The first post-graduate year should be evaluated and strengthened, identifying it more clearly as a psychiatric training year.
12. The RRC should increase its effectiveness in determining standards and monitoring compliance with them.
13. The negative image psychiatry must be challenged at every available opportunity.

Table 1. NRMP PGY-1 Positions Offered/Filled in Psychiatry

Year	Number	Percentage of Total Offered	Percentage Filled by U.S. Graduates	Total
1978	939	5.4	49.6	55.0
1979	966	5.4	45.7	49.9
1980	933	5.2	43.8	47.8
1981	923	5.0	53.0	56.6
1982	922	5.0	58.7	65.4
1983	867	4.8	57.0	70.0
1984	879	4.8	57.0	75.0
1985	902	4.9	66.5	81.9
1986	932	5.0	69.8	83.9

Table 2. Applicants Matching in PGY-1 in Psychiatry Through NRMP

Year	Number of USMGs	Percentage of USMGs	Total Number Matching	Percentage[a]
1978	466	3.9	516	3.9
1979	441	3.6	482	3.6
1980	409	3.3	446	3.3
1981	489	3.8	552	3.7
1982	541	4.2	603	4.0
1983	496	3.9	609	4.0
1984	497	3.7	661	4.1
1985	600	4.4	739	4.5
1986	651	4.1	782	4.8

[a]Total includes FMGs, USFMGs, Canadians, osteopaths, fifth pathway student, etc.

14. Departments of psychiatry should monitor and evaluate the content and methods used to educate primary care physicians about psychiatric illnesses.
15. The American Psychiatric Association should establish a special membership category for medical students.
16. Through more innovative teaching and the increased use of demonstrations, students should see more of what psychiatrists actually do in clinical settings.
17. Efforts should be made to promote small group teaching in psychiatric preclinical courses.
18. Faculty should deal actively with current issues affecting the future practice of psychiatry, including the blurred roles of mental health professionals, third-party insurer discrimination against psychiatric patients, new practice settings, and the effect of neuroscience advances upon the practice of psychiatry.

Many of these recommendations have since been heeded, and implemented. Medical student education in psychiatry has enjoyed greater visibility. Preclinical and clinical courses have become more academically rigorous; recruitment efforts have intensified; many schools have initiated psychiatry clubs; and the RRC has revised its Special Requirements (Essentials) for Residency Training in Psychiatry, tightening the criteria for accreditation of residency programs. Advances in the scientific basis of the field developed through biomedical and behavioral research have had a positive impact on the professional credibility of the specialty.

The APA has joined this effort by establishing a medical student membership category, and by actively advocating that psychiatry improve its public and professional identity as a medical specialty. The results of these activities have been encouraging, as Tables 1 and 2 demonstrate. NRMP and APA census data document the steady increase in American medical students choosing psychiatry; the experiences of department chairmen and residency directors emphasize the steadily increasing quality of these trainees.

6

SELECTION PROCESSES FOR PSYCHIATRIC RESIDENCY

Jerald Kay, M.D.

The diminution of financial support for psychiatric training, the increase in accountability required by government agencies and third-party insurers, the possible surplus of physicians, and the rise of corporate medicine all have had an impact on training. However, the most critical and supraordinate theme addressed by the conference was how best to ensure the educational quality of residency programs. There is no doubt that it is necessary to continue to improve the quality of applicants, assure the quality of training programs, and decrease the variability of educational outcome.

The first of these issues has received considerable attention from concerned groups including the American Psychiatric Association (APA), the Residency Review Committee for Psychiatry (RRC), the American Association of Directors of Psychiatric Residency Training (AADPRT), and the American Board of Psychiatry and Neurology (ABPN). Over the past ten years, there has been a concerted effort to increase the number and improve the quality of medical students recruited into psychiatry residency programs. We have learned that our ability to attract high quality medical students is substantially dependent upon the skill and competence of our residents and faculty.

In 1982, the APA established a Task Force to Study the Quality of Residency Training in Psychiatry. Its mission was to review overall patterns of training, program accreditation, quality of the resident population, and characteristics of the learning experience, funding, resources, and recruitment procedures.

In addressing training program entry requirements, the numbers and qualifications of Foreign Medical Graduates (FMGs), and mechanisms of evaluation and recruitment of future applicants, members of the Task Force expressed concern that the Special Requirements (Essentials) for Residency Training in Psychiatry did not require that FMG applicants demonstrate mastery of basic science and clinical medicine or ensure that only qualified candidates enter psychiatric training programs. The Task Force held that achievement of a passing grade on the ECFMG exam or obtaining a license to practice in the candidate's country of origin failed to provide such assurances.

Subsequently, entry criteria were revised by the Residency Review Committee (RRC), through the Special Requirements (Essentials) for Residency Training in Psychiatry, with similar changes made in the credentialing standards of the American Board of Psychiatry and Neurology. The Special Requirements (Essentials), adopted in 1986, require an Accreditation Council for Graduate Medical Education (ACGME) approved, broad-based year of postgraduate training, with specific experiences in both neurology and the general medical care of patients. The curricula for transferring students must be structured to ensure that all requirements are met during the residency period. Sufficient mastery of English must be demonstrated to ensure accurate, unimpeded communication with patients and teachers.

The new Special Requirements (Essentials) mandate that residency program directors establish a selection mechanism to identify those residents best suited for psychiatric training. Programs also must document application procedures and decision-making processes. Many programs, however, have not yet established formal criteria for admission, allowing their standards to change with the pool of available applicants and the demand for services. These new Special Requirements (Essentials) emphasize the development of standards and, as such, will help to improve the overall quality of residency programs, applicants, and ultimately practicing psychiatrists.

7

ENTRY INTO PSYCHIATRIC RESIDENCY TRAINING: THE PROBLEM CONTINUES

Stefan Stein, M.D.

For many years, psychiatric educators have sought ways to smooth the transition from medical school to residency. Generally, orientation programs have been designed to facilitate the socialization process and help the trainee develop an attitude of openness to learning, a willingness to work, and the trust in the faculty necessary for optimal learning. Inculcation of both professional and ethical standards is often the focus of explicit didactic teaching and individual clinical supervision.

These efforts have been important in assisting the trainee in the transition from student to physician, from generalist to specialist, from onlooker to doer. Socialization, into psychiatry, however, begins earlier. Students see psychiatrists as teachers, supervisors, and models during their medical school years, and their contacts with psychiatrists increase during the process of applying for residency training. How that application process is conducted may affect the residents' approach to their residency programs and their future profession.

Currently, the process of application and acceptance into psychiatry residency training is unregulated by any single administrative mechanism. There is confusion about rules and timing, often leading to misunderstanding and disappointment. Many residency programs do not belong to the National Residency Matching Program (NRMP); some residency programs begin at the second year.

Some of the programs in the Match bend or break rules, demanding commitments or making premature agreements. Students may receive conflicting information from advisors, deans, and the various residency program directors with whom they interview. These experiences cast a negative light on the application procedures, as well as on the specialty.

The Problem

In the early 1960s, the Association of American Medical Colleges (AAMC) adopted a number of rules and procedures to govern medical school acceptance. These recommendations helped decrease the ambiguity that had previously prevailed. In the past twenty years, entry into undergraduate colleges and medical schools has evolved into a well organized system. The procedures are clear, and students are informed in advance of the approximate date on which they will receive notification regarding acceptance. Students also know how much time they will have to make a decision, and when it becomes binding.

In contrast, with the exception of the General Requirements and Special Requirements (Essentials) for Residency Training in Psychiatry, no single mechanism or set of rules exists for residency training programs. The American Association of Directors of Psychiatric Residency Training (AADPRT) is a voluntary organization which includes members from nearly every one of the over 200 accredited psychiatric residency training programs in the United States. It functions largely as an educational resource: convening meetings to facilitate discussion of common problems and serving as a liaison between training directors and other organizations and administrative bodies in medicine and government. It has no authority to enforce rules or regulations. Similarly, the American Association of Chairmen of Departments of Psychiatry (AACDP) is a voluntary membership organization made up of chairmen of all medical school departments of psychiatry. It does not exercise authority over the substance or structure of the total residency training experience, in part, because those residencies not directly affiliated with university departments of psychiatry are not represented in the AACDP.

The responsibility for accrediting residency training programs is held by the Residency Review Committee for Psychiatry (RRC) of the Accreditation Council for Graduate Medical Education. It does not, however, regulate application and selection procedures. It is primarily concerned with the training experience provided once the trainee enters a program.

In 1964, Rosenbaum and Barchilon proposed a mechanism "to appoint residents in psychiatry by a set of rules and regulations...voluntarily agreed upon by some fifty residency training centers" (1). Their plan, a "match" in psychiatry, albeit sound, foundered when the American Board of Psychiatry and Neurology (ABPN) altered the training structure to eliminate the requirement for an "internship" year. At that point, some programs, in order to continue to provide four years of training, arranged for rotations on medical services during the PGY-1. Others, however, maintained a three-year program; this modification required potential entrants to apply separately for appropriate PGY-1 training through the National Residency Matching Program. The result was that two separate systems evolved and even greater confusion occurred.

Today, of the 208 RRC accredited residency programs in general psychiatry, 158 accept trainees only at the PGY-1 level, and 190 accept trainees either at PGY-1 or PGY-2. Not all programs are part of the NRMP.

The Student Applies For Training

In applying for residency training, students must consider a number of variables. Programs vary significantly in size, philosophical orientation, learning experience, and in their link to a university setting, among other variables. The student also must consider such factors as geography and family needs. Students choosing to apply to programs through the NRMP must follow the NRMP calendar requiring submission of preferences by early January with notification in mid-March. This schedule allows little time before the beginning of residency to make necessary arrangements for relocation, job searches for spouses, school placement for children, etc. The NRMP does provide a match for couples, but only if both are in the same year of medical school and wish to be in the same city. Moreover, many of the same students applying for a four-year psychiatry residency also apply to a three year psychiatry residency, interviewing both for a PGY-2 in psychiatry and a separate PGY-1 (e.g., in medicine, pediatrics or a transitional year). Thus, a student may be applying for a PGY-1 position in psychiatry for 1987, a PGY-2 position in psychiatry for 1988, and at the same time, a PGY-1 position in medicine, pediatrics, or family medicine. This complicated arrangement is made worse by the absence of universally agreed upon dates for acceptance into PGY-2 programs or into PGY-1 programs not participating in the NRMP. A student may receive an acceptance from a program which requires a response before NRMP program selections are even made! It is no wonder that program directors and students have developed an oriental bazaar-like system of negotiation.

Discussion and Recommendations

There is no simple, single remedy. Although it can be argued that students do find their way to residencies, the haphazard method is damaging to programs, to applicants, and to the field.

There are a number of options: a PGY-1 and PGY-2 match operated by the NRMP; a separate PGY-2 match for psychiatric programs; a system of single acceptance dates which coincide with the Match, whether the program participates or not. Each solution has advantages and disadvantages. The AADPRT is currently discussing the implementation of a plan with the NRMP. But a reasonable and enforceable system, agreed to by all parties, would be far more desirable than the present situation. It is unlikely that there will be a single administrative body regulating entry into training. It is, therefore, the responsibility of chairmen of departments, training directors, and directors of psychiatric services in hospitals sponsoring training programs, to recognize that compromises are necessary to develop a fair and consistent entry system.

Reference

1. Rosenbaum M, Barchilon J: Toward a unified residency selection plan: Report on a residency selection plan in psychiatry. J Med Ed 39:510-513, 1964

PART 3:

THE RESIDENCY PROGRAM

I. Overview

Residency training programs in psychiatry have significant variability in quality and content, reflecting, at one end of the spectrum, creative use of available teaching resources and clinical sites, and, at the other end, poorly conceived curricula. The conference on training psychiatrists for the 1990s sought to dissect these variations, to analyze training needs, and to make recommendations for the content and structure of future psychiatric residency programs. An introductory chapter describes the state of the field. The issues are segmented into a number of broad headings: Program Planning, Psychotherapy, Research and Technology, Subspecialization, and Evaluation. The chapter authors, participants in the conference, have captured the substance of the debates and discussion. Recommendations are based on consensus-building, and where substantial differences of opinion were registered, they are noted.

Allan Tasman, M.D.
Jerald Kay, M.D.

8

SETTING THE STAGE: RESIDENCY TRAINING IN 1986

Allan Tasman, M.D.

Jerald Kay, M.D.

Before discussing the content and structure of future residency training programs, we will establish the context in which these recommendations are made, the structure and content of present training expeiences, the faculty, and clinical training sites.

The Study

In 1986, a survey was distributed to participants at the annual meeting of the American Association of Directors of Psychiatric Residency Training (AADPRT); a second mailing was sent to non-respondents. The instrument included questions about program size, affiliation, number of full-time psychiatric faculty, and availability of fellowship opportunities. It sought to learn: (1) how much time was devoted to all clinical assignments; (2) at what point in the curriculum were such assignments required; (3) what clinical subjects were offered as free electives or selectives (where residents must make a selection from a restricted list of options); (4) what is the prevailing theoretical model for outpatient psychotherapy instruction; and (5) how many hours per week of classroom teaching and supervision are offered to residents, and how much of that activity is provided by full-time faculty.

Table 1. Clinical Assignments in All Training Programs by Residency Year

Clinical Assignment	Year of Training									Total Programs
	1	2	3	4	5	6	7	8	9	
Med./Ped.	102	0	0	0	0	0	0	0	0	102
Neurol.	69	8	9	3	0	0	0	1	0	90
Inpatnt.	15	19	1	1	67	1	0	2	1	107
Child/Adol.	1	16	52	15	1	8	0	0	3	96
Outptnt.	2	10	49	5	1	13	90	1	8	107
Commun./Psych.	0	5	26	13	0	0	1	0	1	46
Cons./Liais.	0	18	48	0	28	0	3	1	2	100
Alc./Drug	11	11	8	10	0	0	0	0	0	40
Forensic	0	1	12	6	0	0	0	0	0	19
Admin.[a]	0	0	1	24	0	0	0	0	0	25
Elective	1	0	2	90	0	0	0	1	4	98
Emergency[b]	10	15	10	2	2	2	0	0	0	41
Geriat. Psych.	4	3	15	4	0	0	0	0	1	27
Part. Hosp.	0	5	1	0	2	1	0	0	0	9
State M.H.[c]	3	6	1	2	0	0	0	0	1	13
Inpt. Specl.[d]	1	10	6	7	1	2	0	0	1	28
Extend. Psychother.	0	17	8	20	1	5	5	0	8	6

1 = PGY-1 | 4 = PGY-4 | 7 = PGY-2 + 3 + 4
2 = PGY-2 | 5 = PGY-1 + 2 | 8 = PGY-1 + 4
3 = PGY-3 | 6 = PGY-2 + 3 | 9 = PGY-3 + 4

[a]Excludes administrative experiences in PGY-4 offered as electives or chief residencies.
[b]As a specific clinical rotation, not as time on call.
[c]For programs not primarily based at state hospitals or community mental health centers.
[d]Excludes general psychiatric inpatient services.

One hundred and nine of the 208 programs (52 percent) listed in the third edition of the Directory of Psychiatric Residency Training Programs (1) responded. According to the 1984-85 APA census of residents, these 109 programs trained 3,101 residents, or nearly 60 percent of the 5,312 psychiatry residents in the U.S.

Of the responding programs, 77 were located in universities (representing 61 percent of the 126 university programs); 15 were administered by private hospitals (including free-standing psychiatric hospitals); 17 were based at public facilities (state, community mental health center, and military programs).

Faculty included 3,205 full-time psychiatrists, and an even larger number of part-time faculty. The study population demonstrated a trainee to faculty ratio of 0.97, identical to the ratio for programs which had applied for NIMH Comprehensive Institutional Training Grants in the previous fiscal year. Private hospital-based training programs and programs with fewer trainees tended to have lower resident to faculty ratios; higher ratios were found in public facility based programs. Obviously, the psychiatrists had responsibilities (e.g., patient care, research, administration) other than in residency education.

Table 2. Residency Length of Time in Training Programs for Each Clinical Assignment

Clinical	Months of Training								
Assignment	1–2	3–4	5–6	7–8	9–10	11–12	13–24	25–28	Total
Med./Ped.	1	52	37	5	6	1	0	0	102
Neurol.	71	18	1	0	0	0	0	0	90
Inpatnt.	0	2	9	12	13	41	30	0	107
Child/Adol.	5	33	28	0	1	23	6	0	96
Outptnt.	0	2	15	5	4	48	26	8	108
Commun./Psych.	2	15	16	1	1	10	1	0	46
Cons./Liais.	2	42	46	1	2	8	0	0	103
Alc./Drug	29	10	1	0	0	0	0	0	40
Forensic	4	11	2	0	1	1	0	0	19
Admin.[a]	0	8	13	0	0	4	0	0	25
Elective	3	15	29	6	6	35	4	0	98
Emergency[b]	21	11	5	1	0	2	1	0	41
Geriat. Psych.	11	13	2	0	0	1	0	0	27
Part. Hosp.	2	5	1	0	0	1	0	0	9
State M.H.[c]	0	6	4	1	1	1	0	0	13
Inpt. Specl.[d]	2	13	8	2	1	0	3	0	29
Extend. Psychother.	0	2	10	3	0	32	11	0	64

[a]Excludes administrative experiences in PGY-4 offered as electives or chief residencies.
[b]As a specific clinical rotation, not as time on call.
[c]For programs not primarily based at state hospitals or community mental health centers.
[d]Excludes general psychiatric inpatient services.

One hundred and two programs offered four years of training in general psychiatry; the remaining seven maintained three-year residencies, with no PGY-1. While the mean number of residents in the four year programs was 28.5, there was significant variation, ranging from 8 trainees to >80. (Results may not sum to 109. Incomplete or incorrectly reported data were not coded.)

Study Findings

Models of Training

Training directors were asked to describe clinical experiences, including the training year in which they occurred and the percentage of time (rounded to the nearest 25 percent) spent in each. Detailed descriptions of other experiences that did not lend themselves to reporting in the survey's grid format also were elicited.

Survey results indicated that the range of clinical experiences varies widely from program to program. Tables 1 through 4 summarize resident clinical activities in a variety of formats. Table 1 shows that the majority of programs responding required specific clinical experiences in: medicine or pediatrics; neurology; adult inpatient, child and adolescent, outpatient, and consultation-liaison psychiatry. All other clinical activities were required by fewer than half of the responding programs.

Table 2 depicts the length of time a resident is assigned to a particular rotation. In light of growing concern about the apparent increase in the variety of clinical experiences to which a resident is exposed at any one time, the percentage of time spent during each rotation (Table 3) was calculated. As the movement toward specialization in clinical practice evolves, it is likely that simultaneous, multiple clinical experiences will become even more prevalent. In only one clinical training area—inpatient adult psychiatry—do the vast majority of programs train residents more or less full-time, with a significant number of programs including a few hours of outpatient psychotherapy during the rotation. With few exceptions, other clinical experiences are offered on a quarter- or half-time basis.

Table 4 contains the most common responses for length of clinical rotation, percentage of time, and year of training for each clinical activity. The table provides an indication of the manner in which clinical activities are pieced together in each training year.

Table 3. Range of Percentage of Time Spent by Residents in Various Clinical Assignments

Clinical	Percentage of Time						Total
Assignment	5	10	25	50	75	100	Programs
Med. Ped.	0	0	0	0	0	102	102
Neurol.	0	0	1	8	1	80	90
Inpatnt.	0	0	0	2	8	97	107
Child/Adol.	1	3	28	23	2	39	96
Outptnt.	0	0	6	44	19	38	107
Commun./Psych.	1	3	16	13	2	11	46
Cons./Liais.	0	1	13	37	7	44	102
Alc./Drug	0	0	2	3	4	31	40
Forensic	2	1	2	8	0	6	19
Admin.[a]	0	1	0	10	3	11	25
Elective	0	1	6	26	13	51	97
Emergency[b]	0	2	6	8	0	25	41
Geriat. Psych.	0	1	5	6	0	15	27
Part. Hosp.	0	0	2	2	0	5	9
State m.h.[c]	0	1	0	1	0	11	13
Inpt. Specl.[d]	0	0	0	7	3	19	29
Extnd. Psychother.	19	6	31	5	1	2	64

[a]Excludes administrative experiences in PGY-4 offered as electives or chief residencies.
[b]As a specific clinical rotation, not as time on call.
[c]For programs not primarily based at state hospitals or community mental health centers.
[d]Excludes general psychiatric inpatient services.

Table 4. Most Common Responses for Length, Percentage of Time, and Curriculum Year for Clinical Assignments

Clinical Assignment	Length (months)	Percentage of All Programs	Percentage of Time	Percentage of All Programs	Years of Training	Percentage of Programs
Med./ped.	3–4	15	100	100	PGY1	100
Neurol.	1–2	79	100	89	PGY1	77
Inpatnt.	11–12	38	100	9	PGY1–2	63
Child/Adol.	3–4	34	100	41	PGY3	54
Outptnt.	11–12	44	50	41	PGY3	46
Commun./Psych.	5–6	35	25	35	PGY3	57
Cons./Liais.	5–6	45	100	43	PGY3–4	82
Alc./Drug	1–2	73	100	78	PGY1–2	28
Forensic	3–4	58	50	42	PGY3	63
Admin.[a]	5–6	52	100	44	PGY4	96
Elective	11–12	36	100	53	PGY4	92
Emerg.[b]	1–2	51	100	61	PGY2	37
Geriat. Psych.	3–4	48	100	56	PGY3	56
Part. Hosp.	3–4	56	100	56	PGY2	56
State M.H.[c]	3–4	46	100	85	PGY2	46
Inpt. Specl.[d]	3–4	45	100	66	PGY2	36

Note. This table represents the percentage of programs which stated they required this clinical experience, not all programs responding to survey.

[a]Excludes administrative experiences in PGY-4 offered as electives or chief residencies.

[b]As a specific clinical rotation, not as time on call.

[c]For programs not primarily based at state hospitals or community mental health centers.

[d]Excludes general psychiatric inpatient services.

Table 5. Range of Didactic/Seminar Hours per Week by Year of Training

Hours/Week	PGY-1 ($N = 81$)	PGY-2 ($N = 96$)	PGY-3 ($N = 96$)	PGY-4 ($N = 96$)
1	4	0	0	3
2	11	2	2	6
3	11	6	7	9
4	17	18	16	22
5	10	10	13	13
6	9	17	18	17
7	3	2	4	4
8	3	15	9	7
9	2	5	5	0
10	5	8	11	6
11	0	1	1	0
12	3	6	4	3
13	0	1	2	0
14	0	1	0	1
15	2	3	3	0
16	1	1	1	1

Table 6. Range of Supervisory Hours per Week by Year of Training

Hours/Week	PGY-1 ($N = 79$)	PGY-2 ($N = 94$)	PGY-3 ($N = 94$)	PGY-4 ($N = 91$)
1	7	0	1	2
2	13	12	5	8
3	22	17	15	21
4	14	19	20	21
5	10	16	16	21
6	4	12	20	10
7	2	1	4	2
8	1	6	6	4
9	0	0	1	0
10	4	4	1	1
11	0	1	0	0
12	2	4	3	1
13	0	0	0	0
14	0	0	0	0
15	0	0	1	0
16	0	0	0	0
17	0	0	0	0
18	0	0	0	0
19	0	0	0	0
20	0	2	1	0

For most programs, the longest clinical experiences remain inpatient adult psychiatry, and ambulatory rotations with extended psychotherapy training.

Supervision and seminars are the other cornerstones of training. The provision of supervision and didactic experiences across a number of concurrent clinical areas also raises questions about the optimal amount of information trainees can integrate and retain.

Increasing concern about the financial vitality of psychiatric faculty working in academic health science centers (2) prompted inquiry about the time spent by faculty in teaching and supervision (Tables 7 and 8). More than half of the programs reported that full-time faculty are responsible for more than 80 percent of classroom teaching. The largest amount of full-time faculty teaching and supervision occurs during PGY-1. Those programs that do not offer an internship year are at an economic disadvantage.

In later years of training, full-time faculty supervision is distributed bimodally. Half of the programs reported that full-time faculty provide 50 percent or less of supervision; the other half stated that 70 percent of supervision was provided by full-time faculty. Supervision by part-time faculty appears to increase in successive years of the residency programs: in PGY-2, 59 programs reported that 70 percent or more of supervision is provided by full-time faculty; by PGY-3, only 45 programs reported the same level of full-time faculty; and in PGY-4, the number drops to 40 programs. Reliance on part-time and volunteer faculty for didactic teaching and supervision is significant, particularly in the ambulatory setting, and is likely to increase further in the near future.

Clinical Settings

Of the responding programs, fewer than half (46) reported requiring experiences in community settings, and only 13 programs not based at state hospitals or CMHCs reported requiring community clinical experience. The relative dearth of required clinical experiences in community based and public settings often is explained by questions about the suitability of the patient population for a training experience, the adequacy of on-site supervision, the adequacy of ancillary professional staff, and fiscal limitations which complicate or restrict reimbursement to the training program for residents' work on-site. Of course, the same questions should arise in any setting, and their answers should influence resident placement.

Subspecialization

Table 9, abstracted from the Directory of Psychiatry Residency Training Programs, lists a large number of available postgraduate fellowships. Because many of these opportunities are supported by

Table 7. Range of Percentage of Teaching Time by Full-Time Faculty per Year

Percentage of Teaching Time	PGY-1 (N = 77)	PGY-2 (N = 95)	PGY-3 (N = 94)	PGY-4 (N = 89)
5	0	0	0	0
10	3	2	1	1
15	0	0	1	3
20	0	0	0	0
25	0	0	2	2
30	4	5	3	3
35	0	1	1	1
40	1	1	2	2
45	0	1	0	0
50	6	11	14	16
55	0	0	0	0
60	2	3	2	3
65	0	1	1	1
70	0	3	3	3
75	4	8	9	5
80	7	8	16	9
85	0	2	1	1
90	4	13	11	8
95	1	3	2	1
100	45	33	25	30

federal training funds, the future of which is uncertain, it is difficult to predict the future course and availability of fellowships. A move toward increased subspecialty training will require a significant infusion of resources—both personnel and financial—the sources of which are not readily identifiable.

Training in Psychotherapy

Increased demands to integrate rapidly appearing biomedical and behavioral knowledge into residency training, and increasing constraints on psychiatric service reimbursement, have raised concern about the residents' ability to learn to treat patients over extended periods of time. Uncertainties regarding practice setting and patterns, too, have prompted broad debate about the efficacy of psychotherapy training. The emergence of a variety of models of psychotherapy has led to still further debate about the differential use of these psychotherapies, the appropriate model for teaching psychotherapy, and the value of such education. The survey results have suggested that this topic will remain an issue for debate for some years to come.

While many academicians believe that the psychoanalytic or psychodynamic model of psychotherapy has lost its centrality in education programs, 86 of the programs surveyed (79 percent)

Table 8. Range of Percentage of Supervision by Full-Time Faculty by Year

Percentage of Teaching Time	PGY-1 ($N = 76$)	PGY-2 ($N = 93$)	PGY-3 ($N = 92$)	PGY-4 ($N = 87$)
5	0	0	0	0
10	1	2	1	3
15	0	2	4	1
20	0	1	0	0
25	2	2	7	8
30	5	4	5	4
35	0	0	0	0
40	0	1	2	0
45	1	0	0	0
50	3	16	19	23
55	0	0	0	0
60	2	3	7	5
65	2	0	0	2
70	0	2	2	1
75	5	11	14	12
80	5	11	8	4
85	0	0	0	0
90	4	7	7	7
95	0	1	2	1
100	46	30	14	16

Table 9. Programs Offering Post-Residency Fellowships[a]

Area	Percentage	Percentage of All Programs
Administrative	40	19
Alcohol/Substance Abuse	8	2
Biologic/Psychopharmacology	6	2
Child/Adolescent	166	80
Consultation/Liaison	72	35
Family	3	1
Forensic	26	12
Geriatric	40	19
Psychosomatics	4	2
Research	62	30
Student Health	4	4

[a]From 1986 edition of *Directory of Psychiatric Residency Training Programs*, published by AADPRT, AMSA, APA, and SNMA.

identify their predominant outpatient psychotherapy teaching orientation as psychoanalytic (though the descriptions of clinical experiences offered to residents failed to clarify what was meant by this term). Twenty programs cited an eclectic orientation; one recorded a cognitive orientation. Not a single program listed a behavioral therapy approach. Forty-five programs confine outpatient psychotherapy experiences to formal 6 to 12 month rotations.

While teaching may embrace a psychodynamic model, clinical experiences of relatively short duration do not provide the continuity of experience traditionally thought to be essential. The remaining 64 programs offer residents opportunities to treat patients in psychotherapy outside their formal outpatient rotations. Nearly half of these programs permit residents to carry patients for as long as 36 months. Thus, while these data suggest that the core of psychotherapy training utilizing a psychodynamic approach has eroded significantly, the majority of programs still preserve an opportunity for long-term work with patients, despite pressures for limited curriculum time.

Conclusion

Today's residents receive a broad-based education, reflecting the diversity of the field. Predictions are difficult because psychiatric theory and practice are not always in harmony, and training directors cannot predict future clinical practice patterns or sources of financial support. Accredited programs must comply with the Special Requirements (Essentials) for Residency Training in Psychiatry of the RRC by providing specifically identified clinical rotations in medicine or pediatrics; neurology; inpatient, outpatient, child and consultation-liaison psychiatry. Beyond this mandate, however, there is great variability in what residents are taught, by whom, and for how long, as well as where clinical experiences occur. This variation reflects both the philosophy of the individual programs and the availability of local resources. It also illustrates the difficulty in arriving at a consensus for an ideal training model, including defining the appropriate length and type of clinical assignments, and the ideal mix of training in a variety of areas.

References

1. Robinowitz CB, Kay J, Taintor Z: Directory of Psychiatry Residency Training Programs. Washington DC, American Psychiatric Association, 1986
2. Guggenheim FG, Nadelson CC: Earn-as-you-go pressures in academic psychiatry. Am J Psychiat 141:1571-73, 1984
3. American Board of Psychiatry and Neurology, Inc: Information for Applicants. Chicago, IL, ABPN, 1986
4. American Medical Association: Special Requirements of Residency Training in Psychiatry and Neurology. Chicago, IL, AMA, 1986

5. Rudy LS: The psychiatrist and psychiatric education, in Comprehensive Textbook of Psychiatry IV. Edited by Kaplan HI, Sadock BJ. Baltimore MD, Williams and Wilkins, 1985

PART 3:

THE RESIDENCY PROGRAM

II. Program Planning

This section assesses the relevance, efficiency, and vitality of the current instructional cornerstones of residency training: patient care, individually supervised clinical experiences, and didactic seminars. It places the training model in relation to changing practice settings in psychiatry. With psychiatry's rapidly changing knowledge base, it is likely that new training methods or approaches must be developed to ensure quality of clinical care. The forms these should take and the clinical settings for training are not yet clearly defined.

Langsley's initial assumptions provide an overview. He cautions that clinical education should not be governed solely by changes in the health care delivery system, and raises criticisms of both current medical school psychiatry curricula and the traditional psychoanalytic supervision model in residency programs. While advocating the continued centrality of seminars, he argues for the introduction of new educational technology, on which Taintor concurs in his commentary.

Wiener, also agreeing with Langsley, argues against charting new directions in clinical education based primarily on changing practice settings. Drawing again on the distinction that has been made between "education" and "training," he questions the wisdom of prematurely altering training when the practice settings are not necessarily firmly entrenched in the health care delivery system. Wiener also emphasizes that clinical values and ethics are central to university hospital-based training programs, but not necessarily as well defined or emphasized in many new settings governed by "cost containment" principles or a profit motive.

Reading, Fernandez and Shaw, on the other hand, predict the demise of the university teaching hospital as we know it today. They, too, draw the distinction between education as "learning to know," and training, "learning to do," and suggest the latter is highly dependent on where a resident is trained. They remind us that learning is more readily generalized when it takes place in settings comparable to those in which a trainee ultimately will practice. They also argue for the transmission of appropriate attitudes, values, and beliefs, but they provocatively challenge our acceptance of the values of the university setting as more noble ones.

Allan Tasman, M.D.
Jerald Kay, M.D.

9

THE EDUCATION OF TOMORROW'S PSYCHIATRISTS

Donald G. Langsley, M.D.

In discussing the education of tomorrow's psychiatrists, we must make certain assumptions about expected change in psychiatric practice. Clinical training, individual supervision, and didactic seminars have to be placed in this context. Eight assumptions must be highlighted in any discuss of the form and content of future clinical experience, supervision, and didactic training seminars in psychiatric residency.

1. The continuing, rapid expansion of our knowledge base and technology will produce concomitant changes in practice patterns, calling for continuing change in both didactic and clinical education.
2. Psychiatrists will expend more clinical effort in subspecialty areas such as geropsychiatry, forensic psychiatry, clinical psychopharmacology, consultation-liaison psychiatry, and adolescent psychiatry.
3. A smaller proportion of psychiatrists' clinical efforts will be devoted to psychotherapy. Other mental health professionals and paraprofessionals will continue to move into this area, although third-party coverage will become even more constricted than it is today.
4. Psychiatrists increasingly will practice within managed care systems. The psychiatrist, working with a team rather than alone, will act principally as evaluator, treatment planner, consultant, and subspecialist. Other nonphysician professionals will conduct the bulk of psychotherapeutic intervention.

5. Concern about the economics of payment for psychiatric treatment will increase. Today's fee-for-service system will be supplanted not by a fixed-fee, DRG based program, but rather by a fixed-fee system based on capitation or Relative Value Scales.
6. Mechanisms to fund graduate medical education will become more complicated in the wake of declining federal investment in the future supply of physicians as a whole and of subspecialists in particular. Federal funding for subspecialty education is already changing, and will continue to do so, increasingly affecting primary residency training. Reimbursement to residents for the services they provide patients will be emphasized.
7. The number of foreign medical graduates (FMGs) entering training will be further reduced. Some states are already placing limits on FMG funding; others are refusing licenses to FMGs. Entry and licensure examinations for FMGs have become more rigorous, and a new clinical skills evaluation will be required for entry into U.S. graduate medical education programs. Plans to require accreditation of off-shore medical schools, where many U.S. citizens now obtain substandard medical education, may force some schools to close. Public facilities which now depend heavily upon the FMG pool will reanalyze their medical manpower needs and readjust their hiring patterns.
8. Performance evaluations will gain prominence, not only during residency, but also in certification, recertification, and the determination of hospital privileges. Salaries also may become dependent upon such evaluations.

While psychiatrists still practice psychotherapy as one of their professional activities, this skill no longer sets the psychiatrist apart from other practitioners. Psychiatry is now one of several mental health professions engaged in the practice of psychotherapy. If anything distinguishes the psychiatrist from nonphysician mental health professionals, it is the medical skills acquired during residency. These integrate medical knowledge with a thorough background in the biopsychosocial determinants of behavior, the capacity to do broad-based evaluation and treatment planning for the mentally ill, and the authority to prescribe and carry out certain medical treatments.

Basic Psychiatric Education/Training

Education, as has been noted in previous chapters, refers to the processes whereby the student develops judgment, problem-solving ability, creative modes of thinking, an appreciation of the questions to ask, and the skill to identify medical assumptions and evaluate them critically (Tables 1 and 2). Training, a set body of knowledge and skills to be mastered by the future practitioner, includes attention to all the basic biopsychosocial aspects of psychiatry, and also must focus on scientific thinking, both by critical analysis of the literature and by participation in research.

The current approach to psychiatric training, which consists of clinical experience with individual supervision and didactic seminars, will remain the core of residency training. What will and must change are the means and settings in which these core experiences will be taught. To remain static, to suggest that psychiatric education need not change, is to fly in the face of reality. The challenge is to predict the future with a precision which will enable us to make changes in psychiatric education.

Clinical Experience

In all medical specialties, a major locus of clinical experience has been the hospital. Psychiatry led other specialties in moving substantial portions of clinical education into the outpatient clinic, to the emergency room, and to the community. As has been noted, current trends in the organization of health care delivery, however, will require future specialists to be taught to work both in managed care systems such as Health Maintenance Organizations (HMOs) and in vertically integrated, investor-owned systems.

Table 1. Critical Skills

Comprehensive interviewing
Evaluation of need for hospitalization
Capacity to be reliable and maintain integrity in practice
Diagnostic accuracy
Treatment plan formulation and implementation
Assessment of suicidal or homicidal potential, or potential for assaultive behavior
Provision of supportive psychotherapy with awareness of dynamic issues
Effective use of psychopharmacological agents
Mastery of maintaining interest in, tact, and compassion for patients
Recognition of both contertransference problems and personal idiosyncrasies
Recordkeeping

Table 2. Critical Knowledge

Criteria for differentiating organic and functional processes
Indications and contraindications for common psychopharmacological agents
Characteristics of and explanations for various psychiatric disorders
Differential diagnosis of psychiatric syndromes
Evaluation and management of psychiatric emergencies
Indications and contraindications for hospitalization and other interventions
Descriptive psychiatry
Genetic and dynamic formulations
Principles of human growth and development
Theories of therapy
Specific syndromes of importance in consultation psychiatry
Psychotherapies: psychoanalytic psychotherapy

Though the acute care hospital will continue as the basic locus of learning about inpatient psychiatry, other settings also will remain part of the resident's clinical experience. The outpatient clinic, including its extensions into the community, will continue to be a major site for residency education, but it will expand its focus so that long-term dynamically oriented psychotherapy will no longer be the predominant clinical experience provided there.

As has been indicated, the status of psychotherapy continues to remain high in most residencies. Programs that focus on dynamic psychotherapy emphasize outpatient rather than inpatient experience. The general psychiatrist normally engages in office-based psychotherapy, with a small amount of time devoted to hospital consultation or direct care. Seventy percent of psychiatric time is devoted to psychotherapy. As increasing numbers of nonphysician practitioners engage in psychotherapy, will residencies place as great an emphasis on mastering this skill? Can and should this modality be maintained as a central skill of the residency program if fewer practicing psychiatrists are engaged in psychotherapy?

The move toward subspecialization also will have an effect upon the locus of clinical experience. The most significant implication of subspecialization is the development of specialized clinics and service programs for geriatric patients, forensic problems, consultation-liaison psychiatry, etc. The approach is not dissimilar to those subspecialization models found in internal medicine, pediatrics, and obstetrics/gynecology, in which these specialized clinics and inpatient services are the locus of at least some residency training.

Psychiatry resembles other medical specialties in its rapid movement toward a series of subspecialties. We already have recognized specialized training in child psychiatry and in psychoanalysis. Child psychiatry now has fellowships, accredited training programs, and certification mechanisms. Increasing numbers of psychiatrists, however, are focusing on other subspecialties, the majority of which are not as well-developed as child psychiatry. These include: forensic psychiatry, which has developed its own certification process outside the American Board of Psychiatry and Neurology (ABPN), administrative psychiatry, substance abuse, and geropsychiatry. Other fields which may become subspecialties include adolescent psychiatry, clinical psychopharmacology, and consultation/liaison psychiatry. Without ABPN development of certification mechanisms for these areas, those involved in geriatric psychiatry and other emerging subspecialties will surely develop their own certifying boards as has forensic psychiatry.

Individual Supervision

Clinical instruction in medicine has long been based upon a one-to-one model. Such an approach calls on the teacher to demonstrate the necessary clinical skills, and to be available for the important psychological processes of identification and modeling. Clinical skills are not learned predominantly from books or video demonstrations; they are understood and assimilated by exposure, observation and practice. The finer points of examination, interviewing, problem-solving, and decision-making are best taught by interaction.

The majority of clinical disciplines approach such teaching from a "bedside" model. The teacher "rounds" with the students, hears about the history and findings, and may then perform certain types of examination to demonstrate the necessary problem-solving skills to the students. The same kind of interaction, demonstration, and discussion occurs in the operating room, the laboratory, or the clinic. Clinical problem-solving involves interaction between teacher and student, and the clinical skill of the teacher is what engenders the highest respect from students. The learning process involves a high degree of identification. Although medical students have more actual contact with residents than with senior faculty, students seem to find their most valuable educational experiences with faculty, rather than with the residents who serve more as older siblings than as parents.

Psychiatry has adopted a somewhat different approach, with supervision based on the psychoanalytic educational model where reports of patient sessions are brought to the supervisor's office, and both the trainee and supervisor try to understand the events from these reports. The length, frequency, and intensity of psychoanalysis make it impossible to check for consistency and repetition. The working-through process almost guarantees that there will be multiple review opportunities. The candidate is often an experienced psychiatrist, having completed a psychiatric residency, several years of personal analysis, and some course work; the patient is generally relatively healthy and able to verbalize. This model seems to work well for the psychoanalyst.

Unfortunately, this approach has many limitations as a model for basic psychiatric residency training. The intensity, frequency, and length of the brief or supportive psychotherapy in which a resident engages may vary significantly from those of psychoanalysis and do not lend themselves to the same check and review process. The patient population is more diverse and not necessarily as healthy or verbal. The student is not as experienced a clinical psychiatrist as is the analytic candidate, and the supervisor is often not as skilled in various models of care delivery. Our trainees often come to value dynamic formulations regardless of whether the formulations apply to the specific patient.

In the past, our clinical teaching process also differentiated psychiatry from other medical disciplines. Instead of using rounds, where patients are seen by attending-teaching staff and students, psychiatric staff often did little more than review history and patient charts. Efforts "not to dilute the transference" or "to maintain confidentiality" could lead to a failure to interact with the patients. The student did not see the teacher actually deal with the patient.

Recent technological advances have introduced technical methodology such as closed-circuit television to psychiatric education. Videotaping patients allows both student and teacher to view interactions, although it does not substitute fully for face-to-face involvement among patient, student, and teacher.

In many psychiatric residencies, students still cannot watch a teacher "in action" except during conferences. Such participation cannot substitute for direct observation of the conduct of therapy or similar professional activities.

Didactic Seminars

By the 1990s, teaching techniques will be affected profoundly by advances in educational technology. Computers will be used increasingly for instruction and self-assessment; the addition of videotape/videodisc interactive technology will provide excellent clinical simulations. Electronic communication will permit students engaged in clinical rotations away from the home residency program to participate in didactic seminars and to receive consultation on-site.

The National Board of Medical Examiners is developing a series of examinations employing this new technology. Candidates may take an exam using a microcomputer connected to an interactive videodisc. Simulated clinical problems require the physician to conduct a diagnostic evaluation and initiate and maintain clinical management, as is done in practice. The computer will record every action taken by the physician or student, permitting assessment of quality of care, cost, risk, and decision logic.

Technology also may assist in didactic instruction. Students may be taught by "master teachers" though separated by hundreds of miles. A library of routine and unusual "cases" to be reviewed as needed will expand greatly the student's knowledge base.

These new electronic networks cannot substitute for teachers, journals, books, and face-to-face interaction, but they can enrich traditional approaches.

In sum, the core of psychiatric education will continue to emphasize clinical experiences, coupled with individual supervision and broadened by didactic seminars. The framework may be modified to include the ever-changing new knowledge base, through use of technology.

References

1. Langsley DG: Today's teachers and tomorrow's psychiatrists: Presidential address. Am J Psychiat 138:1013-1016, 1981

2. Langsley DG, Hollender MH: The definition of a psychiatrist. Am J Psychiat 139:81-85, 1982

3. Langsley DB, Yager J: Proposal for subspecialties in psychiatry. Unpublished monograph, 1986

10

FUTURE RESIDENCY PROGRAMS WILL BE RICH IN CONTENT

Zebulon Taintor, M.D.

While future residents will continue to glean important patient information from the clinical diagnostic interview, their diagnostic armamentarium also will include sources beyond those signs and symptoms elicited in face-to-face patient intercourse. These include data derived from laboratory and other tests, as well as from assessments of a patient's longitudinal history.

Diagnostic data relating to drug abuse, toxic psychoses, and many DSM-III Axis III disorders are currently derived from urine, blood, and cerebrospinal fluid analyses. In the 1990s, it is possible that a typology of the schizophrenias and major affective disorders may emerge based on receptor measurements in such peripheral fluids. Similarly, numerous high-technology, mechanical innovations, such as brain electrical activity mapping (BEAM), magnetic resonance imaging (MRI), and positron emission tomography (PET) are becoming more widely accessible. In the 1990s, residents will learn to make highly focused diagnoses based upon these and other advances in brain electricity and body imaging, that will further unravel the vast complexities of brain functioning.

Equally important will be increasing emphasis on sophisticated assessment of the longitudinal history of the patient. Residents in the 1990s will be focusing more extensively on the chronic patient and will have increasing numbers of tools available either to reconstruct a patient's longitudinal case history or to access sources of that information. As noted in earlier chapters, the computer may be of significant assistance, enabling psychiatrists to retrieve existing patient records more readily, and also helping to gather pertinent information directly from the patient.

As a resident's clinical experiences will be broadened by the use of these new techniques, so too will supervision be changed. One-to-one supervision is limited by the knowledge base of the supervisor. The field is growing faster than individual faculty learning, thus defining the limits of individual supervision and emphasizing the need to consider new teaching alternatives for the 1990s and beyond. The innovative use of peers, group supervision, and self-study techniques (often computer-aided) may to help bridge the gap between supervisors' limits and the knowledge to be gained by the resident. Similar to the group learning in didactic seminars, which is dependent upon collective synthesis of knowledge, the use of these new supervisory techniques will provide a level of group supervision and feedback greater than the sum of its parts and substantially beyond that available in the traditional one-to-one supervisor-resident relationship.

Computer-assisted learning—through instant books, bulletin boards, literature retrieval services, among others—will play a major role in residency knowledge acquisition in the 1990s. Didactic seminars will be "team taught" to overcome the gaps in individual trainer capacity to keep current with the field. Peer didactics, too, will gain favor, with more senior residents providing their junior colleagues with the benefit of their insight and experiences.

Throughout residency training, however—whether through clinical experience, supervision, or didactic seminars—people, not technologies, will remain central. The increased availability of electronic texts will not substitute for the interaction and affect generated in seminars or lectures. Self-assessment or clinical experience cannot be expected to replace entirely the relationship of student to supervisor. The competency to use sophisticated diagnostic equipment may make assessment decisions more certain, but alone cannot substitute for the careful evaluation of the patient's function, signs, and symptoms through the clinical interview.

11

THE ROLE OF UNIVERSITY TEACHING HOSPITALS IN FUTURE TRAINING AND PRACTICE

Jerry M. Wiener, M.D.

Should psychiatrists be trained to "meet the needs" of those specific practice settings most likely to be prevalent in the coming decade? If the response is in the affirmative, does this mean that the university teaching hospital is a wasteful, less productive setting in which professionals are trained to function in ways that may be irrelevant to the future? The answer to each of these questions is an emphatic "no."

These questions are based on a series of fallacious assumptions deriving from the failure to address two simple concepts: "patient" and "education."

The first assumption is that physicians—psychiatrists—should only be "trained," and that the training should be tailored specifically to fit the shape and needs of settings, not those of patients. The emphasis is on the development of expedient skills, the capacity to ply a trade, and not upon knowledge and principles, the cornerstone of a profession.

Psychiatry is a profession, a medical specialty for which an education with empirical and theoretical knowledge is at least as important as the acquisition of skills. The physician also must acquire a set of attitudes and ethical standards, learned through interaction with teachers who also serve as role models. It is not clear whether debate and discussion, communication of knowledge, theory, clinical wisdom and experienced judgement, and the challenge of entertaining different perspectives will be valued and supported in newer treatment settings.

By extension, it may be an implicit assumption that patient needs for diagnostic assessment, biopsychosocial formulation, and appropriate treatment recommendations will vary by setting, and further, that patient needs will be subordinated to the needs of the setting. For example, although the typical Health Maintenance Organization (HMO) "mental health" benefit covers up to 20 outpatient visits and 30 inpatient days per year, administrators may disallow claims by the way in which an illness is defined. Thus, if an illness is considered chronic or not susceptible to improvement within the covered service period, benefits may be disallowed. The determination to disallow claims or discontinue treatment based upon chronicity or lack of potential improvement may depend upon the needs of the setting to hold down costs and to improve patient flow, not upon the needs of patients seeking care. Psychiatrists in such settings can be caught in a conflict between their medical and ethical responsibility to patients and their contractual relationship with their employer.

Should the education and training of psychiatrists—or of any physicians—be defined or limited to what an insurer will reimburse? If so, critical questions of ethical compromise are raised, especially about the care of patients requiring long-term intervention.

Another implicit assumption is that training can and should be provided in sites divorced from, uninterested in, or even alien to the multifaceted interplay between the training/educational process and research, scholarship, and interaction with mentors in psychiatry and across specialties. There is no disagreement that, in fact, training can occur in less intellectually oriented environments. However, the psychiatrist of tomorrow must be an expert in the understanding, diagnosis, formulation, and treatment of mental illnesses within both a pluralistic theoretical model and a broad array of therapeutic modalities. With this complex knowledge base, psychiatrists may become equally knowledgeable and skillful in applying that learning to patients encountered in a variety of service systems.

Service delivery sites may well have a variety of conditions, special circumstances, and even restrictions within which psychiatric care can be provided. Those psychiatrists who choose to work in such settings (and their number will likely increase) will be expected to adapt and function effectively within requirements or limits, and in keeping with the needs of their patients. The capacity to work within such constraints is not likely to be acquired by training tailored strictly to the needs of the service system alone.

Still another fallacious assumption is that the university hospital is an anachronism, not a relevant setting for patient care, compared to the alternatives. The university hospital is a reality-oriented institution, rapidly adapting to survive, and, most important, to fulfill its primary missions of quality care in support of education and training objectives. Under its auspices, aspects of education and training can and probably should be undertaken in alternative practice sites, but not to the exclusion of the university hospital itself.

Psychiatric educators and practitioners alike recall the excitement in the 1960s and 1970s when the community mental health movement was seen as the vanguard of future psychiatric practice. Many programs answered this siren's song, shifting major training functions to the community mental health centers, only to founder on the rocks of indifference or antagonism to the priorities and costs of training. With past as prologue, it seems unlikely that the new service settings of the 1990s will be more congenial learning environments than were the community mental health centers of past decades. Given the emphasis upon cost containment and restricted benefits, HMOs seem unlikely sites for psychiatric trainees to learn how to care for the severely mentally ill. Neither the for-profit corporate hospital nor the emergency care center seems any more likely as a future training program of excellence. While public sector outpatient and chronic care units beckon, our trainees may be faced with a system that is chronically underfunded, poorly staffed, and leeched of morale by the responsibility of caring for the most severely ill under very adverse circumstances.

The answer must lie with our university hospitals. Yet, their future is in jeopardy. Today's university-academic health center may not remain adaptively competitive as a health care delivery system, able to offer a balance of quality and cost-effective care that patients and, more important, payers will continue to buy. Because professional education and clinical training can take place only where there are patients, the question becomes not whether we should shift our training, but whether we will be forced to do so.

While the jury is still out on this last question, it does appear that the university health center will prevail. Certainly, there may be increasing compromise including ancillary training sites at HMOs, rotations through for-profit inpatient and emergency facilities, and care for chronic patients at public hospitals. However, the priorities and values of the university hospital residency program are such that the field and the quality of patient care would be greatly impoverished if our next generation of psychiatrists do not have the advantage of such an education.

12

CHANGING PSYCHIATRIC TRAINING SETTINGS IN THE '90s

Anthony Reading, M.D.

Robert C. Fernandez, M.D.

Kailie Shaw, M.D.

University teaching hospitals, as we know them, will probably cease to exist in the 1990s. Like the great dinosaurs of the past, they will prove to be too large and cumbersome, too inflexible, and too narrowly adapted to survive in a rapidly changing and increasingly competitive environment (1). Academic hospitals of the 1990s will have to focus on patlent care as their first responsibility, if they are to attract appropriate patients for their teaching and research programs (2). To ensure economic survival, these hospitals will have to be organized to provide the types of medical care and services that their communities need, rather than simply address the specialized interests of their faculty.

Given the increasing number of highly competitive specialist graduates entering practice, often in the same community, university teaching hospitals will no longer be able to count on a monopoly for referrals for prestige care or for complex procedures. Clinical teaching in the 1990s will occur where the patients are. In psychiatry, increasingly patients will be in Health Maintenance Organizations (HMOs), small general hospitals, private for-profit mental hospitals, public sector outpatient and chronic care units (3).

As a result, selected representatives of these types of institution will become the university teaching hospitals of tomorrow. Teaching residents to practice psychiatry, as has been stated in previous chapters, involves both education and training. Education is relatively independent of the circumstances in which it occurs, while training is much more dependent upon the setting in which it is conducted. There is a wealth of educational theory and research that supports the common sense notion that the carry over of learning from one situation to another is directly related to the degree of similarity between the settings (4). We tend to forget that the context of learning can be as important as the content in determining whether it will be accessible in another setting. Many in academic psychiatry are familiar with medical students who function most capably on a psychiatric rotation, but who are not able to think "psychosocially" during medicine or surgery rotations. If the setting in which a skill is acquired differs significantly from the one in which it will be applied, the skill may not be transferable.

To the extent that future settings in which psychiatry will be practiced will differ significantly from current university teaching hospitals—in patient type, range and severity of illness, care models and organization, resource constraints, etc.—these traditional facilities will not adequately prepare trainees for practice in the 1990s. To educate psychiatrists for the diversity of practice patterns that will characterize the next decade, we must assist them to develop a greater variety of skills in a greater range of settings than they have had in the past. We must teach them how to apply knowledge to the patients they will see in the future and in the settings that will exist.

We are not advocating that all of our current university teaching hospitals simply be closed down and their trainees sent out into the world to complete their education. Applied training sites do differ from ordinary community practice settings. Teaching facilities need resources to support their educational activities. Universities will have to take the lead in setting up teaching units in the practice settings that they believe will be relevant to the future (5). To succeed, these units will need to be intellectually stimulating bases for applied research that appropriately reward their faculty. One of the growing challenges facing academic psychiatry as it moves into the 1990s will be how to become more effective in bridging the gap that exists between theory and practice. The changes underway in medicine represent an unprecedented opportunity for universities to venture out from the security of the ivory tower, to bring the best of modern psychiatry into community settings.

Still, training involves more than just the acquisition of skills and knowledge. Patterns of future practice depend a great deal on the professional values, attitudes, and beliefs acquired during training. Trainees absorb the culture, viewpoints, language, customs, and beliefs of the "families" in which they are raised. We must be able to foster a view of the future with optimism and convey a positive image of psychiatry.

The changes taking place present an opportunity for academic psychiatry to integrate itself better with practice. The gulf between academia and the practice community continues to be a barrier to the effective transfer of new knowledge. We need to sensitize our trainees in vivo to the realities of psychiatric practice, and act s appropriate clinical role models for them. As psychiatry changes, so should the training and training sites. These new settings can become the university teaching hospitals of tomorrow. We need to espouse them and what they stand for with enthusiasm, to commit ourselves and our resources to them fully, to study and improve them, to make them centers of inquiry and excitement, and to see them as the challenges and opportunities that they are.

References

1. Schwartz WB, Newhouse JP, Williams AP: Is the teaching hospital an endangered species? NEJM 131:157-162, 1985
2. Petersdorf RG: Is the establishment defensible? NEJM 309:1053-1057, 1983
3. Reading A: Involvement of proprietary chains in academic health centers. NEJM 313:194-197, 1985
4. Ellis HC: The Transfer of Learning. New York. McMillan Co., 1965
5. Warren JV, Plumb DN, Trzebiatowski GL, eds.: Medical Education for the 21st Century. Columbus OH, Ohio State University College of Medicine, 1985

PART 3:

THE RESIDENCY PROGRAM

III. Psychotherapy

Few topics galvanize our field in quite the manner of the debate on the role of psychotherapy in the future conduct of clinical psychiatric practice. Considerable controversy was generated during the Raleigh Conference about the appropriate place of psychotherapy, and particularly-long term psychotherapy, in teaching and practice for the future.

This issue arises, in part, because of the tension about the growing amount of "bio" and shrinking amount of "psychosocial" in the biopsychosocial training model over the past two decades. Increasing pressure has been placed on the curriculum to make room for the rapidly increasing knowledge base, especially in the neurosciences. Unless the training period is lengthened, we will soon reach the limits of our curriculum time; we may find that we must set priorities and decide which clinical experiences we can reduce or do without. One of the clinical experiences to be considered by those setting priorities for training curricula is long-term psychotherapy.

Recently, there has been pressure to examine the role of long-term psychotherapy in comparison to short, highly structured treatment modalities upon which research and outcome studies have recently focused. The absence of studies of long-term psychotherapy from the outcome literature and the absence of reports of indications for this form of therapy have led some to advocate its elimination from the training curriculum. In addition, public policy makers, third-party payers and others have raised questions about the efficacy of long-term psychotherapy and the role of the psychiatrist in rendering such treatment. Further, competition from other mental health disciplines has led to debate about psychiatry's unique or different role in providing such care, particularly when it is of long duration.

The papers by Simons and Tucker lay a foundation for many of the issues related to psychotherapy in residency training. They raise or imply a host of questions:

1. *How is one trained/educated for psychological understanding? Is there any route other than by doing psychotherapy?*
2. *What is meant by "psychotherapy"? Is this term equivalent to psychoanalytic psychotherapy? Is the teaching value of traditional, psychoanalytically oriented psychotherapy based on its duration, its intensity, both, or neither?*
3. *Are residents trained only to be skilled technicians?*
4. *Is anything beyond good interviewing skills really necessary for a psychiatrist to deal with the interpersonal issues that arise in the care of patients?*

Tucker forcefully poses the central questions in his evocative paper, arguing against the notion that future psychiatrists should be trained as competent psychotherapists. He believes that this issue is an "historical question, asked primarily by those who are locked into a period of time." Tucker traces the prominence and promise of psychoanalytic theory and practice in America; he questions the ethics of such prolonged treatments in the absence of efficacy data. Psychotherapy is linked provocatively with treatment of the "worried well" to the exclusion of those suffering from severe, chronic mental disorders. He suggests that the focus of DSM-III upon phenomenology and diagnosis, coupled with the increasing "demand for precision and specificity in our practice" argue against the continued centrality of psychotherapy. His forecast is that tomorrow's psychiatrist will be predominantly a consultant with broad-based knowledge, but substantially less expertise in psychotherapy. Tucker forsees other mental health professionals providing the bulk of psychotherapy services.

On the other hand, Simons suggests that competency in psychotherapy will remain an essential part of residency training. Central to his approach is a six dimensional model that integrates biological, psychological, sociocultural, and descriptive aspects with tradi-

tionally psychoanalytic dynamic and developmental genetic perspectives. The latter two are important, Simons posits, to explain how and why a given mental disorder arose through current and past life experiences. He provides an excellent and cogent summary of recent psychotherapy research focusing on the relationships among therapist and patient, the agents of therapeutic change, and the nature of transference.

The debate calls into question many of the basic assumptions held by those who have developed training curricula in the past; it raises nearly as many questions as answers. Yet, in the end, it suggests a tightly circumscribed role for psychotherapy training as part of the core residency curriculum.

Allan Tasman, M.D.
Jerald Kay, M.D.

13

THE ROLE OF PSYCHOTHERAPY IN PSYCHIATRIC EDUCATION

Richard C. Simons, M.D.

To question the role of psychotherapy as a critical ingredient of a residency training curriculum suggests a misperception of the nature of psychiatric practice. During the first half of this century, the explosion of knowledge from psychoanalysis led many to conclude that the appropriate treatment approach for all mental disorders must be based on a psychodynamic model. The decade of the 1960s saw a similar enthusiasm for the social psychiatry model, reflected in the community mental health movement. Now we have come full circle. With the revolution in biological psychiatry of the past decade, many psychiatrists believe that the treatments for the future must be the biological therapies.

The etiologies of most (if not all) of the mental disorders are multiple, involving biological, psychological, and sociocultural determinants. The treatment of these disorders, then, should involve biological, psychological, and sociocultural modalities, as envisioned in George Engel's biopsychosocial model (1, 2). The ability to function as a competent psychotherapist is essential in order to achieve these optimal diagnostic and treatment goals.

Evaluation of the Psychiatric Patient

The diagnosis of psychiatric patients has been approached from a variety of perspectives in order to integrate biological, psychological, and sociocultural factors with descriptive, dynamic, and developmentalgenetic diagnostic models.

Table 1. Evaluation of the Psychiatric Patient[a]

Models	Descriptive	Dynamic	Developmental-Genetic
	Physical exam		
Biological	Current physical strengths Current physical disorders or conditions (DSM-III Axis III)	Biological factors in mental illness	History of genetic and other constitutional factors History of physical illness, injuries, operations, medications
	Mental status exam		
Psychological	Current psychological strengths and adaptive functioning (DSM-III Axis V) Presence of one or more mental disorders (DSM-III Axis I and Axis II)	Psychodynamic factors in mental illness Learning factors in mental illness	Developmental factors and experiences in infancy, childhood, adolescence, and adulthood
	Life setting		
Sociocultural	Current psychosocial supports (DSM-III Axis V) Current psychosocial stressors (DSM-III Axis IV)	Sociocultural factors in mental illness	Family history Racial, religious, cultural, and socioeconomic background

[a]Table by Richard C. Simons.

Our current nosology of mental disorders, exemplified by DSM-III, utilizes the descriptive model (3). DSM-III describes what strengths and liabilities are present in any given patient using five different axes. Axes I and II focus on the diagnosis of any present mental disorder. Axis III addresses current physical disorders and, by implication, current physical strengths as well. Axis V emphasizes current psychological strengths and adaptive functioning of the patient, while Axis IV provides an assessment of current psychosocial stressors in the patient's life.

The dynamic model attempts to explain not what, but *how* a given mental disorder has come about, by assessing the present interaction of multiple etiological factors—biological, psychological, and sociocultural. The developmental-genetic model attempts to explain *why* a given mental disorder has arisen, as the result of *past* interaction of biological and environmental factors. Each of these dimensions must be taken into account in order to achieve, first, a full diagnostic assessment and then, a rational and effective treatment plan.

An Overview of the Psychiatric Therapies

Just as the biopsychosocial approach is used to evaluate a patient, it may be used to conceptualize distinctions among the psychiatric therapies, which can be divided into three categories: the biological (somatic), the social (environmental), and the psychological (4).

The pharmacotherapies are the predominant biological therapies in use today. Social therapies attempt to make positive alterations in the patient's environment, and include hospitalization with milieu therapy, day treatment, occupational therapy, creative arts therapy, residential placement, support groups, and sheltered workshops. Psychological therapies may be described by reviewing their theoretical underpinnings, their treatment context, their duration, or their goals. If conceptualized on the basis of a specific theoretical model, therapies would cluster around the psychodynamic models, learning theory models, and existential models, among others (5). Contextual distinctions would include individual, group, marital or family therapy; duration would cluster around crisis intervention, short-term and long-term therapy. Therapeutic goals would be based on supportive, symptom-oriented, or insight-oriented approaches.

Psychoanalysis, thus, would be considered one of the individual psychotherapies in which the long-term goal is to achieve meaningful insight into and resolution of chronic intrapsychic and interpersonal conflicts that cannot be addressed effectively by short-term approaches. Crisis intervention, on the other hand, provides immediate symptomatic relief from acute distress. Whatever the model, context, length of treatment, or goal, the same factors are critical outcome predictors: (1) the therapist's contribution to the therapeutic relationship; (2) the patient's contribution to the same relationship; (3) the nature of the therapist-patient interaction; (4) the agents of therapeutic change; and (5) the nature of the transference.

Current Trends in Psychotherapy Research: An Overview

It is beyond the scope of this paper to attempt a systematic review of the complex field of psychotherapy research, but it is appropriate to recognize the advances made in the past decades in systematic investigation of the factors influencing the outcomes of psychotherapies (6-14). Convincing data are beginning to emerge supporting the importance of the five factors cited above as significant outcome predictors.

Therapist, Patient, and Therapeutic Relationship

Hartley recently reviewed research on the therapeutic alliance in psychotherapy, including the therapist's contribution, the patient's contribution, and the interaction between the two (15). In the same volume, Luborsky and Auerbach focused on the same factors in a review of 85 studies of psychodynamically oriented psychotherapy (16). They found that:

1. About 70 percent of these studies show a significant ability to predict treatment outcomes.
2. Relationship factors are more highly predictive than patient or therapist factors.
3. Within the relationship factors that are most often predictive are measures of the helping alliance and the match of the patient with the therapist.
4. The results apply both to psychodynamically oriented psychotherapy and to closely related forms of psychotherapy.
5. When the entire group of 85 studies is divided into short-term and longer-term psychotherapies, two major differences appear: patient factors are likely to be more often significantly predictive in studies of short-term therapy, while the therapist and relationship factors are more often predictive in studies of longer therapies.

Further, a number of studies have provided evidence supporting the view that within an accepting therapeutic relationship, a patient can find the support necessary to trust another human being (17-23). That trust enables the patient to experience realistic hope for the future and to develop "a positive helping alliance with the therapist" (20). Within that alliance, the patient and therapist can work toward the goals of the therapy. While it may be necessary to introduce biological and social therapies to achieve those goals, the competence of the psychiatrist as a psychotherapist will be an essential factor in the success or failure of all therapies employed. As Luborsky has suggested "...the therapist's ability to form an alliance is possibly the most crucial determinant of his effectiveness" (23).

The Agents of Therapeutic Change

Karasu has reexamined whether unique (specific) or common (nonspecific) factors are responsible for therapeutic effectiveness (24). He identified three therapeutic change agents that he believes are shared as underlying bases by all schools of psychotherapy: (a) affective experiencing; (b) cognitive mastery; and (c) behavioral regulation. Affective experiencing is defined as "arousing excitement and responsiveness to suggestion; unfreezing and expression of feelings." Cognitive mastery incorporates "acquiring and integrating new perceptions and thinking patterns, [and] promoting self-awareness and understanding"; behavioral regulation involves "learning and modifying behavioral responses, [and] managing and controlling actions and habits." Karasu concludes by posing three new areas for future research in psychotherapy: 1) techniques that facilitate each of the three change agents; 2) the match between change agents and particular diagnostic subgroups; and 3) the relationship between particular change agents and the therapist-patient dyad. His conceptualization of change agents and future research will allow us to study the actual psychological techniques that lead to change without regard to the particular theoretical construct within which they are utilized.

The Nature of Transference

One of the most exciting developments in psychotherapy research is the attempt to verify the psychoanalytic concept of transference, a universal phenomenon, and one that operates in all therapeutic relationships without regard to orientation. Luborsky pioneered this research, beginning with his established "core conflictual relationship theme method" (CCRT) (25, 26).

In this approach, judges score narrative episodes about relationships that patients describe during psychotherapy sessions. Three components are identified within each episode: the patient's main wishes, needs, or intentions toward the other person in the narrative; the responses of this other person; and the responses of the self. The most frequent of each of these components constitutes the CCRT. Most recently, Luborsky has reported data from the CCRT method related directly to a number of Freud's observations about transference (27, 28). These include: "(a) each patient has one main transference pattern; (b) it is specific for each patient; (c) it applies to love relationships in a broad sense; (d) part of it is located in one's awareness and part is kept out of awareness; (e) the pattern remains consistent throughout a person's life; (f) it can change some; (g) the relationship with the therapist reflects the pattern; (h) the pattern derives from the relationships with the early parental figures; and (i) it is also active in relationships outside of psychotherapy" (27).

Psychotherapy in Perspective

This discussion of the nature, structure, and research understanding of the psychotherapies is intended to provide the framework for discussion of the continued value of psychotherapy training for future psychiatrists. We should avoid nihilism or despair regarding our ability to measure outcome in psychotherapy and our ability to predict the efficacy of various psychiatric therapies for particular mental disorders. We are on the horizon of just such precision and specificity. The teaching of psychotherapy to future psychiatrists will be grounded in scientific reliability and validity as well as in the rich tradition of clinical observation and experience.

Functions Performed by Training in Psychotherapy

Training in psychotherapy is essential to our ability to diagnose a wide range of mental disorders, and then to offer the appropriate psychiatric therapies to patients. The Group for the Advancement of Psychiatry Committee on Therapy has described three of these functions:

> *[W]e can identify at least three functions that are performed by training in psychotherapy. First, a set of skills based on a body*

of knowledge is taught, one that is indispensable to becoming a practicing psychotherapist. True, not all psychiatry residents will become psychotherapists. Yet, these skills in understanding and dealing with distressed people are necessary for the optimal practice of other modalities of therapy, such as pharmacotherapy or behavior modification therapy. Examples would be the ability to perceive that a schizophrenic patient may stop taking medication in response to fears of engulfment or in an attempt to be returned to the hospital with its nurturant care, and the knowledge to predict that a patient may respond more readily to one program of 'shaping' behavior than to another, because it offers more opportunity to identify with the therapist. Second, the process of psychotherapy itself acts as a vital laboratory for the acquisition of essential knowledge. An attempt to teach psychodynamics without psychotherapeutic experience is equivalent to an attempt to teach human anatomy without dissection. One can describe phenomena to a student, but he cannot see and experience them for himself—an essential pedagogical requirement. Third, training in psychotherapy facilitates a set of attitudes. These attitudes include:

1. *A readiness to attend to all aspects of individual communicative behavior, including covert as well as overt, paralinguistic and kinesic as well as linguistic, and omissions or apparent irrelevancies as well as relevant content.*
2. *A readiness to adopt a nonjudgmental attitude of attentive, "active," empathic listening and observation in the face of a wide range of feelings in the patient.*
3. *A readiness to employ one's own evoked emotional responses as sensitive diagnostic tools.*
4. *A readiness to consider multiple and hidden motivations to account for behavior.*
5. *A readiness to consider and integrate a patient's transference attitudes and responses into a total therapeutic plan, regardless of the therapeutic modality employed.*
6. *A readiness to consider a patient as a whole person within a biopsychosocial context, whose suffering is to be alleviated without undue compromise of autonomy. Although family and general practitioners are returning to the once commonplace awareness of the patient as a whole person, nowhere else but in psychiatry is the value of the patient's autonomy taught so explicitly and with such emphasis.* (29)

The goals of psychotherapy, therefore, are at the center of the experiences presented in our residency programs.

Conclusion

In *Heart of Darkness*, Joseph Conrad wrote, "The mind of man is capable of anything—because everything is in it, all the past as well as all the future" (30). Surely, the diagnostic assessment of any psychiatric patient must do justice to this richness of the human mind and spirit, this capacity for good as well as evil, this complex interaction between strength and vulnerability. Once we have made a diagnostic assessment, our treatment approaches must be directed to the patient's needs, not the clinician's interests or the researcher's theories. Yager's goal of "enlightened eclecticism" (31) is not only laudable, but actually attainable. According to this goal, each clinical situation is viewed from multiple theoretical perspectives, and those treatment approaches are then selected which most closely address the patient's needs and wishes, without sacrificing the best information available.

Marmor made the point clear when he warned against the fallacies of biological, psychological, and sociological reductionism, and urged instead "an awareness of the pluralistic, multifactorial origins of psychopathology" that "broadens our understanding and increases our therapeutic potential" (32). More recently he has noted: "One fact seems increasingly clear. We can no longer bow to the sectarianism that loudly asserts the superiority of one psychotherapeutic technique over all others. An 'enlightened eclecticism' that encourages therapists to employ a biopsychosocial approach to understanding the disturbances in the patients' life-systems, and adapt their techniques accordingly, points the way to further developments in individual psychotherapy" (33).

Similarly, the future of psychiatric education, clinical practice, and research rests on integration, not fragmentation. Future psychiatrists must be trained as competent psychotherapists to be able to integrate and implement all of the biological, psychological, and social therapies at their command with increasing precision, specificity, and effectiveness. As the GAP Committee on Therapy has concluded: "Only by respecting the complexity and pluralism of modern psychiatry and neither exalting nor depreciating psychodynamics and psychotherapy will the increasing polarization within our field be reversed and the values of psychodynamic sensitivity, as well as psychotherapy, enrich all of psychiatry" (29).

References

1. Engel GL: The need for a new medical model: A challenge for biomedicine. Science 196:129-136, 1977
2. Engel GL: The clinical application of the biopsychosocial model. Am J Psychiat 137:535-544, 1980
3. American Psychiatric Association: Diagnostic and Statistical Manual of Mental Disorders, 3d Ed. Washington DC, American Psychiatric Association, 1980
4. American Psychiatric Association Commission on Psychiatric Therapies, TB Karasu, Chairman: The Psychiatric Therapies. Washington DC, American Psychiatric Press, 1984
5. Karasu TB: Psychotherapies: An overview. Am J Psychiat 134:851-863, 1977
6. Kernberg OF, et al: Psychotherapy and psychoanalysis: Final report of the Menninger Foundation's psychotherapy research project. Bull Menninger Clinic 36:1-275, 1972
7. Luborsky L, et al: Comparative studies of psychotherapies: Is it true that "everyone has won and all must have prizes"? Arch Gen Psychiat 32:995-1008, 1975
8. Luborsky L, et al: Predicting the outcome of psychotherapy: findings of the Penn Psychotherapy Project. Arch Gen Psychiat 37:471-481, 1980
9. Smith ML, Glass GV, Miller TI: The Benefits of Psychotherapy. Baltimore MD, Johns Hopkins University Press, 1980
10. American Psychiatric Association Commission on Psychotherapies, TB Karasu, Chairman: Psychotherapy Research: Methodological and Efficacy Issues. Washington DC, American Psychiatric Association, 1982
11. Karasu TB: Recent developments in individual psychotherapy. J Hosp Comm Psychiat 35:29-39, 1984
12. Williams JBW, Spitzer RL, Editors: Psychotherapy Research: Where Are We and Where Should We Go? New York, Guilford Press, 1984
13. Wallerstein RS: Forty-Two Lives in Treatment. New York, Guilford Press, 1986
14. Luborsky L, et al: Psychotherapy: Who Will Benefit and How? The Factors Influencing the Outcomes of Psychotherapy. New York, Basic Books (In Press)
15. Hartley DE: Research on the therapeutic alliance in psychotherapy, in American Psychiatric Association Annual Review, Volume 4. Edited by Hales RE and Frances AJ. Washington DC, American Psychiatric Press, 1985, pp. 532-549

16. Luborsky L, Auerbach AH: The therapeutic relationship in psychodynamic psychotherapy: the research evidence and its meaning for practice, in American Psychiatric Association Annual Review, Volume 4. Edited by Hales RE and Frances AJ. Washington DC, American Psychiatric Press, 1985, pp. 550-561
17. Gomes-Schwartz B: Effective ingredients in psychotherapy: Prediction of outcome from process variables. J Consult Clin Psychol 46:1023-1035, 1978
18. Marziali E, et al: Therapeutic alliance scales: Development and relationship to psychotherapy outcome. Am J Psychiat 138:361-364, 1981
19. Moras K, Strupp HH: Pretherapy interpersonal relations, patients' alliance, and outcome in brief therapy. Arch Gen Psychiat 39:405-409, 1982
20. Morgan R, et al: Predicting the outcomes of psychotherapy by the Penn Helping Alliance Rating Method. Arch Gen Psychiat 39:397-402, 1982
21. Luborsky L, et al: Two helping alliance methods for predicting outcomes of psychotherapy: Counting signs vs. a global rating method. J Nerv Ment Dis 171:480-491, 1983
22. Buckley P, et al: Psychodynamic variables as predictors of psychotherapy outcome. Am J Psychiat 141:742-748, 1984
23. Luborsky L, et al: Therapist success and its determinants. Arch Gen Psychiat 42:602-611, 1985
24. Karasu TB: The specificity versus nonspecificity dilemma: toward identifying therapeutic change agents. Am J Psychiat 142:687-695, 1986
25. Luborsky L: Measuring a pervasive psychic structure in psychotherapy: The core conflictual relationship theme, in Communicative Structures and Psychic Structures. Edited by Freedman N and Grand S. New York, Plenum Press, 1977, pp. 367-395
26. Luborsky L: Principles of Psychoanalytic Psychotherapy: A Manual for Supportive-Expressive (SE) Treatment. New York, Basic Books, 1984
27. Luborsky L, et al: A verification of Freud's grandest clinical hypothesis: The transference. Clin Psychol Rev 5:231-246, 1985
28. Luborsky L, et al: Advent of objective measures of the transference concept. J Consult Clin Psychol 54:39-47, 1986
29. Group for the Advancement of Psychiatry Committee on Therapy: Teaching Psychotherapy in Contemporary Psychiatric Residency Training. New York, GAP, 1987

30. Conrad J: Heart of Darkness (1902). New York, Bantam Books, 1969, p. 60
31. Yager J: Psychiatric eclecticism: A cognitive view. Am J Psychiat 134:736-741, 1977
32. Marmor J: Systems thinking in psychiatry: Some theoretical and clinical implications. Am J Psychiat 140:833-838, 1983
33. Marmor J: Psychotherapy: Releasing the dark, transparent stream. J Hosp Comm Psychiat 35:5, 1984

14

PSYCHOTHERAPY WILL NOT BE CENTRAL IN PSYCHIATRIC EDUCATION

Gary J. Tucker, M.D.

Whether psychiatrists should be trained as competent psychotherapists is a question asked primarily by those locked into a particular period of time, and it is answered best by an historical perspective. Prior to World War II, psychiatric practice in the U.S. was centered in state hospitals. The model psychiatrist either worked in a hospital or, if in private practice, was primarily a consultant with extensive psychiatric and neurologic training. During World War II, a large influx of European psychoanalysts brought with them a treatment that offered the hope of curing mental illness. The promise offered by psychotherapy, particularly psychoanalytic psychotherapy, resonated with the intellectual and emotional climate of that era. A hope was held out that with enough time, skill, and money, mental illness would be treated and personalities would be restructured. In its brief, forty-year life in the history of American psychiatry, psychoanalytic psychotherapy has become more pervasive than in any other medical community in the world.

However, in the past ten to fifteen years, many forces have conspired to deemphasize the role of psychotherapeutic approaches in psychiatric practice. Psychotherapy always has been a treatment for those with financial means—whether personal wealth or generous insurance benefits. It has not fulfilled its promise either for the masses or for those suffering with serious mental illness.

Moreover, it has raised questions about the benefits and the cost of prolonged intensive psychotherapy.

Data bearing on the efficacy of this modality have been scant, in part because this form of treatment does not fit into a traditional medical model. It is difficult to delineate the indications, the dose, the side effects, the adverse effects, and the end point. In this context, attention has turned to more specific and quantifiable therapies such as behavioral and pharmacologic interventions.

With the rise in the use and demonstrated effectiveness of psychopharmacologic agents, further questions about the efficacy of psychotherapy began to be raised. At the same time, increasing emphasis has been placed on the diagnostic process itself, as treatments appear to be specific for particular diagnoses. DSM-III, the culmination of this more specific diagnostic approach, is helping to return psychiatry to a more medically oriented model; toward biology, away from speculation and introspection, and toward a clear demand for precision and specificity in practice.

The march of medical knowledge itself has conspired against psychotherapy. Twenty years ago, almost the entire didactic curriculum was related to psychotherapeutic interventions. There was little taught on the diagnostic process or on the biologic aspects of mental illness. Today, training programs have great demands placed on them to include not only new data about biological psychiatry, but also about community psychiatry, social networks, psychoeducational approaches, forensic issues, ethics, families, etc. In short, a substantially greater body of knowledge is being conveyed to our trainees today, and, concomitantly, psychotherapeutic training has diminished as the core of residency training.

Some may argue that these are not good reasons to abandon a treatment. However, if psychiatry is to assume some role in the care of the seriously mentally ill, and not just the "worried well," we must continue to emphasize other treatments in our training programs. Psychotherapy as the major province of the psychiatrist is of historical interest and has little pertinence for our future.

Even if we could all agree that every psychiatrist should be "trained as a competent psychotherapist," we would have to come to some agreement about which psychotherapeutic theories would be included in our training curriculum. There is no common definition of psychotherapy. A 1985 gathering in celebration of the 100th anniversary of the opening of Sigmund Freud's consulting offices was described as "the greatest concentration of psychotherapeutic talent to gather in one place since Freud dined alone.... It showed what these 100 years have wrought: a babble of conflicting voices" (1).

The search for a general description of psychotherapy leads to oversimplification, as in this definition offered by Jerome Frank:

> *Psychotherapy may be viewed as an influencing process that has emotional, cognitive and behavioral facets. Emotionally it tries to produce and maintain a degree of arousal optimal for learning, to foster hope, self-confidence, and trust, and to combat despair, insecurity, and suspicion. Cognitively, psychotherapy helps the patient to achieve new and more accurate understanding of his problems and ways of dealing with them. From the behavioral standpoint, it requires that the patient participate in some form of activity that leads to behavioral changes outside the therapeutic situation.* (2)

This very general definition describes many interactions that physicians, religious leaders, politicians, and the military have used for centuries. Psychotherapy is an undefinable treatment that has gained its status because it has been used by a high status figure—the physician/psychiatrist. In part, Frank goes on to make the same case when he states:

> *The psychiatrist's status as a physician enables him to inspire confidence in his patients and to strengthen their self-esteem through his acceptance of them. Some psychiatrists, in addition, have undergone analytic training, which teaches a particular body of doctrine linked to a special technique, affords extensive experience in the use of the method, and includes an analysis of the trainee. This training has many values, including mastery of an inclusive and penetrating theory of human nature and enhancement of the analyst's self-knowledge, but the superiority of analytic treatment over other methods remains to be demonstrated. This suggests that part of the popularity and persistence of analytic training may lie in its effectiveness as an indoctrination procedure. In this connection, similarities of analytic training to thought reform are pointed out.* (2)

Such sociologic explanations may explain the persistence of psychotherapy in our psychiatric residency curricula. Certainly, on the basis of efficacy we cannot claim hegemony for any one psychotherapeutic theory in which we must inculcate all of our trainees. In a paper subtitled "Is It True That Everyone Has Won and All Must Have Prizes?" which reviewed controlled studies comparing psychotherapies, Luborsky found insignificant differences among psychotherapeutic interventions (3).

When we have no data demonstrating the primacy of any one type of psychotherapy, the development of a curriculum that adopts a particular school of psychotherapeutic theory seems thoughtless, at best. Before we can require training in a particular area, we must develop criteria defining that area. Psychotherapy, to date, has not been so defined.

Moreover, we must set aside the misguided assumption that, absent psychotherapeutic training, a psychiatrist will not gain competence in interviewing skills and psychologic understanding. Every psychiatrist should be trained as a competent interviewer and should have an awareness of the dyadic interaction. The skills may be taught within any number of therapeutic approaches, and across any number of settings, and are not solely the province of psychotherapy.

Frank places psychotherapy within this broader context of adjunct therapies, recognizing its role as part, but not the whole of psychiatric care when he characterizes the physician-patient relationship as:

> *A circumscribed, more-or-less structured series of contacts between the healer and the sufferer, through which the healer, often with the aid of a group, tries to produce certain changes in the sufferer's emotional state, attitudes, and behavior. All concerned believe these changes will help him. Although physical and chemical adjuncts may be used, the healing influence is primarily exercised by words, acts, and rituals in which the sufferer, healer, and, if there is one, group, participate jointly.* (2)

What Frank argues for is a balance among approaches to the treatment of a patient. Equally, we must be more balanced in our approach to the role of psychotherapy in our residency training curricula. In the 1960s and 1970s, psychopharmacologic agents were seen as symptomatic treatments; physicians who used them were "avoiding" or "distancing themselves" from intimate, direct patient contact. The use of medications would only "cover up" the need for "real treatment" to change the personality structure in the psychotherapeutic setting. While the medical model, to which we have returned, may be of greater benefit in the rehabilitation of the seriously mentally ill, we have recognized that the biological revolution has not yet fulfilled its promise. While reductionism persists, most training programs and psychiatrists have turned to an "eclectic" and pragmatic approach that matches treatment to patient, balancing biologic and psychologic interventions.

This is not to suggest that psychiatrists should not become expert in psychotherapy. Rather, those who seek expertise should engage in such training after the completion of their residency, much as psychiatrists interested in child and adolescent, geriatric or administrative expertise do. It is clear that the days of the centrality of psychotherapy training in our residencies are over. It is equally clear that one does not have to be a psychotherapist to be a competent psychiatrist.

Our residency training program curricula should reflect this newfound theoretical freedom from domination by the psychotherapeutic model.

References

1. Krauthammer C: The twilight of psychotherapy. The Washington Post, December 27, 1985
2. Frank J: Persuasion and Healing. Baltimore MD, Johns Hopkins Press, 1961
3. Luborsky L, Singer B: Comparative studies of psychotherapies: Is it true that 'everyone has won and all must have prizes?' Arch Gen Psychiat 32:995-1008, 1975
4. Detre T, Tucker G: Psychotherapy for the mentally ill: a redefinition of goals, in The New Hospital Psychiatry. Edited by Abrams and Greenfield. New York, Academic Press, 1971, pp 57-65

PART 3:

THE RESIDENCY PROGRAM

IV. Training for Research/Technology

There can be no future for a field that does not develop a research base to enhance its clinical efficacy. Psychiatry must invest in its future. The scientific advances in our field over the last few decades have been spectacular, and this forward momentum must be sustained. Pincus, in his chapter, reviews the state of research in psychiatry, including the need to increase the number of skilled researchers and the fiscal constraints imposed upon them. He suggests approaches to the recruitment and retention of talented researchers and defines the scope of preparation necessary for research careers, as well as the supports that sustain productivity.

The same growth of knowledge and technology that brings forth new directions in clinical care also creates new teaching and training opportunities. In their chapter, Fidler and Robinowitz describe the need to integrate the new technologies of computers, video technology, and telecommunications into both the form and content of psychiatric training curricula, and suggest how these new approaches may be used to enhance training, evaluation, and clinical practice.

Carol C. Nadelson, M.D.
Carolyn B. Robinowitz, M.D.

15

RESEARCH TRAINING IN PSYCHIATRY: CURRENT ISSUES AND FUTURE NEEDS

Harold Alan Pincus, M.D.

Opportunities for research in psychiatry have never been as abundant or exciting as they are today. Although powerful new scientific technologies can be applied to investigate psychiatric disorders, increasing constraints on the field have given rise to grave concern about our ability to apply these new developments (1, 2). Foremost among these constraints is the impact of chronic underfunding for mental and addictive disorder research, with federal research funds currently amounting to less than 0.5 percent of the direct treatment costs of these disorders (1-5).

Equally important are questions regarding the adequacy of the research expertise of today's psychiatrists. The current pool of skilled psychiatric investigators is insufficient, and as research continues to expand, the need will continue to grow (1, 6). This chapter examines the supply and demand for properly trained clinical investigators and suggests a broad-based approach for developing future clinician-researchers in psychiatry.

Issues

That there are insufficient numbers of clinical researchers is a problem not unique to psychiatry. Commentators have raised concern about the "dwindling bedside connection" of all medical research, as fewer medical students and residents are motivated to enter academic and research careers (7, 8). Describing the physician-investigator as an "endangered species," Wyngaarden has documented the dramatic decline in interest in research, in participation in research training programs, and in the proportion of National Institute of Health (NIH) grant awards to faculty with M.D. degrees (9).

For psychiatry, the impediments to research careers have been more serious and of longer standing (10-13). In 1967, the Group for the Advancement of Psychiatry noted that "psychiatric investigation has yet to become a widely established part of the profession" (10). Two decades later, that critique remains valid, despite enormous research accomplishments in the intervening years. The majority of research activities are limited to a small core group of academic departments (6). Nearly half of the nation's psychiatry departments are without a single research grant award from the National Institute of Mental Health (NIMH); about 77 percent of all NIMH grants are awarded to just 10 percent of the departments. This concentration of research funding, and, consequently, research programming, in a few centers has increased in recent years. Although it may be inevitable, and even quite desirable to have a core group of "centers of excellence," the dramatic, growing concentration suggests that relatively few medical students have any exposure to research-intensive experiences in psychiatry.

Equally alarming is the evidence that, in general, psychiatry faculty have little specialized training in research. In the 1983 National Academy of Sciences report on biomedical and behavioral research personnel needs, a comparison of psychiatric faculty and those in general medicine (including internal medicine, family practice, obstetrics-gynecology, and dermatology) showed that fewer members of psychiatric departments had research training or experience than in the other specialties surveyed (14). Thirty-four percent of the M.D. faculty in general medical departments had at least one year of post-doctoral research training, whereas only 12.4 percent of psychiatric faculty had that level of research training. Two-thirds of medical faculty members participated in some research, but only about half of psychiatric faculty were similarly engaged. Thirteen percent of all M.D. faculty were Principal Investigators on an NIMH or ADAMHA research grant, contrasted with only 4.5 percent of psychiatry faculty (14).

To address these findings, it is useful to consider our capacity to locate, educate, and maintain a new generation of clinician-researchers.

Recruitment

While the field seems to have reversed the decline in the percent of medical students entering psychiatry, the number of those interested in research careers remains only a fraction of the number coming into the field. It is essential that we attract medical students with the greatest scientific interest, talent, and ambition.

A key factor in fostering interest in research is early exposure, either in medical school or college (15, 16). Mechanisms to provide such exposure, however, are often regarded as an expensive frill, not an essential focus for education. With the majority of scientific activities being conducted within relatively few research-intensive departments, we need to develop more systematic mechanisms to expose a broader array of students to research experiences.

Financial disincentives also impede recruitment. While the question of remuneration over the course of a research career is of concern, a more immediate obstacle to recruitment is the cost of medical education itself. Confronted with an amassing debt, many students are reluctant to seek low-paying summer research fellowships that would provide early involvement. Residents, too, are reluctant to consider one- or two-year fellowships for more intensive research training after they have completed their residency. Over the past six or seven years, a steadily diminishing proportion of NIMH research grants have been awarded to younger scientists (i.e., those under 36 years of age) (17). The implications of this trend are ominous, particularly as established, senior investigators begin to phase down research activities.

Women psychiatrists also are markedly underrepresented in research (18). While women represent 19.5 percent of all psychiatrists, only 6 percent of NIMH research grants to psychiatrists had female principal investigators. We need to consider possible disincentives to the choice of research career paths for women psychiatrists. Since women now represent nearly 40 percent of psychiatric residents, these issues will become even more critical in the future.

An extensive and sophisticated recruitment effort is necessary to produce sufficient numbers of qualified researchers, including:

1. Increasing psychiatrist-researchers' awareness of their unique potential to interest medical students and residents in research careers (19). Enthusiastic successful role models can help convey to students the extent of career satisfaction and excitement (20).

2. Having psychiatry departments identify a "research recruitment coordinator" to promote student recruitment systematically, to provide a clearinghouse and to match students with research opportunities, to provide counseling and support, and to seek funding to support these efforts (21).
3. Developing and expanding opportunities, particularly for medical students, to be involved in an intensive research experience. The recently implemented NIH-Howard Hughes Medical Institute program, providing senior medical students with a 6-month to one year training program in an NIH laboratory, has tremendous potential for influence. Psychiatry departments should make specific efforts to identify and assist students who might be candidates for this program. Further, psychiatric research centers should consider the development of extramural programs based on this model (19).
4. Requiring all residents to have an experience in planning and/or conducting empirical research. This experience, appropriately supervised, should include: critical literature review, hypothesis development, data acquisition plans (including comparative review of relevant instruments), data analysis plans (including statistical analysis), inferences, limitations and conclusions. Ideally, actual data collection should be part of the experience (14, 22).
5. Establishing a formal track for residents interested in research careers, in research-intensive departments of psychiatry. Such departments could serve as regional resources collaborating with other departments in their geographic area to enable interested and qualified residents to pursue these tracks.
6. Emphasizing the recruitment of women (18) and minorities (23), and eliminating the disincentives to their pursuit of psychiatric research careers.

Preparation

In-depth scientific training is essential for almost all research, and psychiatric research is no exception. Certainly, such a program would be useful. However, the notion that a Ph.D. "is necessary to do good research is incorrect and unfortunate" (24).

A number of models exist to train physicians, including psychiatrists, as clinical investigators (5, 25, 27-30). These models vary in site and support, including federal research centers, medical schools that are privately or federally funded, and foundation funded training such as the Robert Wood Johnson Clinical Scholars Program, the Markey Fellowships, Pfizer Scholars, etc. All include

common features such
at least two years; ong
mentor; presence in a
for research support.

While maintaining a
cian, programs must p
special role of the clin
tation to science; (b)
objective questions; (c)
atic inquiry in either
values of scientific med

Research training sho
psychiatry (e.g., biologi
vestigators for the full
ticular needs stand out:
apy research), health se
schizophrenia, substance abuse, and most notably, child psychiatry.

In order to achieve these goals, academic psychiatrists must be willing themselves to train further in research. One of the unfortunate distinctions between teaching psychiatrists and other academic physicians is the lack of research experience within our profession based, in part, on the generalist orientation of the field. Academic physicians in other specialties, such as internal medicine, are likely to have completed subspecialty fellowships, the majority of which require research experience. Only rarely are they generalists. Psychiatry's primary subspecialties—child and forensic psychiatry—remain clinical skills oriented, and do not provide substantive research training. Thus, the challenge is to train not only residents, but many of their teachers, to the nature and conduct of psychiatric research.

Retention

A related issue is our ability to sustain and nurture career aspirations. Young clinical investigators typically complete a two-year research fellowship, then face three or more years as junior faculty. In that capacity, they carry commitments to undertake research, teaching, clinical services, and administration; they spend up to 30 percent of their time writing grants, many of which end up "approved but unfunded" (31). Further, they accept a relatively low salary compared to the income of their colleagues in private practice. As might be expected, the turnover rate is high (31). Having "served their time," a large number of junior faculty members become discouraged and opt to take advantage of their "golden parachute" into clinical practice.

There are numerous spurs that sidetrack or derail research talent. Among these is the encroachment of administrative and clinical responsibilities. Investigators typically don't function as independent clinical scientists until age 35. Then, if highly regarded, he or she is likely to be recruited for senior administrative positions by age 40 or 50, leaving a narrow "career window" for productive research.

Research career development must be seen as an ongoing process in need of continued stability, maintenance and renewal.

The Role of the Mentor

In *The Oddyssey*, Homer gives the name *Mentor* (steadfast and enduring) to the friend Odysseus entrusted with the guidance and education of his son, Telemachus. Levinson has described the essential role of a mentoring relationship in the formative years of a young professional's career:

> *The mentor relationship is one of the most complex, and developmentally important a man can have in early adulthood.... He [the mentor] may act as a teacher,...sponsor,...host and guide,...exemplar,...(and) he may provide counsel and moral support... The mentor has another function, and this is developmentally the most crucial one: to support and facilitate the realization of the Dream. The true mentor, in the meaning intended here, serves as an analogue in adulthood of the "good enough" parent for the child.* (32)

Anecdotal stories also abound regarding the importance of mentor relationships in the career paths of eminent people in the domains of art and literature, sports, as well as science. In fast-moving, highly competitive fields such as scientific research, the role of the mentor can be particularly significant.

Most attention has been paid to the effect of a mentor on a young person entering a career. Not as much attention has been paid to the mentor, per se, to identify those qualities most important for successful fulfillment of that role. There is a need to better assess the number and quality of research trainees working under particular mentors. Psychiatry must find ways to develop and reinforce individuals with those mentoring qualities.

Social Supports and the Reward System

The growth of the basic neurosciences has fostered a community of scientists that offers nurture and social support for younger researchers. Until recently, no similar community existed for clinical scientists in general, and for those with social or behavioral research interests in particular. The absence of such a system has deprived clinical investigators of a certain amount of psychological and social sustenance, and of a collective base upon which to advance. This deficit is being addressed both through the development and increasing visibility of professional societies in these areas, and through concerted efforts to encourage professional interaction among clinical researchers.

Yet, questions remain. How does the presence or absence of mechanisms and policies for advancement, affect the field? To what extent are clinical scientists disadvantaged by the absence of indices of accomplishment specific to their field in competing with basic scientists for funds, tenure, and recognition? How do the complex of administrative, teaching, and clinical demands affect potential advancement? What are the effects of publishing standards and measures on those engaged in psychiatric research? How do competition and the reward system in biomedical science affect the ethical practices and concerns of clinical researchers?

Psychiatric researchers also must recognize that their roles include some "marketing" (30) to the public to develop and expand their currently limited base of support. They should establish regular and frequent lines of contact with elected representatives and public policy makers. Communicating does not imply pandering to popular whim, reductionism, or sensationalism. Academic elitism or aloofness may be more dangerous than honest, if occasionally unsuccessful, attempts to communicate with policy makers.

Impact of Federal Programs

The federal research training programs of the Alcohol, Drug Abuse and Mental Health Administration (ADAMHA) have had enormous impact on the development of research training in psychiatry. While there is cautious optimism that the serious underfunding of research on mental disorders is being slowly corrected, concern continues about the instability of federal support. The Research Career Award and Research Scientist Award programs have been praised for having a major impact on the field (11), and new programs supporting younger researchers such as the Physician Scientist Awards and the First Independent Research

Scientist Trainee (FIRST) Awards, are most welcome. At the same time, it is important that the Agency clearly communicate the nature and rationale for these programs to medical students and residents, and that the programs be flexibly implemented, closely monitored and fully evaluated by the Agency.

A particular concern has been the lack of support for the training of psychiatrists under the National Research Service Awards Act (NRSA). Of approximately 1,000 trainees supported by the NIMH under that program in 1985, only 69 were psychiatrists (33). While the low stipend level had been a disincentive for participation of psychiatric trainees and departments, the increase in stipends to a level commensurate with residency levels has not had a significant positive effect. NIMH is presently undertaking a serious review of research training efforts. We hope it will address this serious and dramatic imbalance.

Conclusion

There is an interdependence among training, research, and the future of psychiatry. Research does change training curricula and practice. Breakthroughs in biomedical and behavioral research also have changed the perception of psychiatry by both the public and public policy makers. Crucial to the balance in this interdependent relationship, however, is the training of future generations of psychiatric investigators. Psychiatry must address a number of challenges—the personal issues affecting the career choices of young scientists, role and socialization into the research community, and issues deriving from the "politics" of academia and government—to ensure our research future.

References

1. Institute of Medicine, Board on Mental Health and Behavioral Medicine: Research on Mental Illness and Addictive Disorders: Progress and Prospects. Washington DC, National Academy Press publication No. IOM-84-08, October 1984
2. Pincus HA, Pardes H: The Integration of Neuroscience and Psychiatry. Washington DC, American Psychiatric Press Inc, 1986
3. Freedman DX: Research funds are down—take heart! Arch Gen Psychiat 42:518-522, 1983
4. Pardes H, Pincus HA: Challenges to academic psychiatry. Am J Psychiat 140:1117-1126, 1983

5. Pincus HA, West J, Goldman H: Diagnosis related groups and clinical research in psychiatry. Arch Gen Psychiat 42:627-629, 1985
6. Burke JD, Pincus HA, Pardes H: The clinician-researcher in psychiatry. Am J Psychiat 143:968-975, 1986
7. Frederickson DS: Biomedical research in the 1980s. NEJM 304:509-517, 1981
8. Cooper JAD: Manpower resources for research. Ann Intern Med 89 (Part2):806-808, 1978
9. Wyngaarden JB: The clinical investigator as an endangered species. NEJM 301:1254-1259, 1979
10. Group for the Advancement of Psychiatry: The Recruitment and Training of the Research Psychiatrist. Report 65. New York, GAP, 1967
11. Boothe BE, Rosenfeld AH, Walker EL: Toward a Science of Psychiatry: Impact of the Research Development Program of the National Institute of Mental Health. Monterey CA, Brooks-Cole Publishing Co., 1974
12. Stein M: Psychiatrists' role in psychiatric research. Arch Gen Psychiat 22:481-489, 1970
13. Report to the President of the President's Commission on Mental Health, Vol 1. Washington DC, US Government Printing Office, 1978
14. Institute of Medicine, National Academy of Sciences: Personnel Needs and Training for Biomedical and Behavioral Research: Publication IOM-83-03. Washington DC, National Academy Press, 1983
15. Bickel J, Morgan TE: Research opportunities for medical students: An approach to the physician-investigator shortage. J Med Ed 55:567-573, 1980
16. Davis WK, Kelley WN: Factors influencing decisions to enter careers in clinical investigation. J Med Ed 57:275-281, 1982
17. Pincus HA: Issues in clinical research in psychiatry, in Clinical Research Careers in Psychiatry. Edited by Pincus HA and Pardes H. Washington, DC, American Psychiatric Press, 1986
18. Nadelson CC, Coffey B, Gean MP: Incentives and disincentives influencing the choice of clinical psychiatric research careers by women, in Clinical Research Careers in Psychiatry. Edited by Pincus HA and Pardes H. Washington DC, American Psychiatric Press, 1986
19. Hillman BJ: The inadequacy in the number and quality of physician researchers: A perspective and approach to the problem. Invest Radiol 20:767-771, 1985

20. Lefkowitz RJ: Not necessarily about receptors. Clin Res 31:543-549, 1983
21. Thier SO, Morgan TE: The other medical manpower problem. NEJM 301:1283-1285, 1979
22. Strauss GD, Yager J, Offer D: Research training in psychiatry: A survey of current practices. Am J Psychiat 137:727-729, 1980
23. Parron DL, Lawson WB: Minorities in clinical research in psychiatry: A challenge for the future, in Clinical Research Careers in Psychiatry. Edited by Pincus HA and Pardes H. Washington DC, American Psychiatric Press, 1986
24. Littlefield JW: The need to promote careers that combine research and clinical care. J Med Ed 61:786-789, 1986
25. Goodwin FK, Roy-Byrne P: Research careers in biological psychiatry, in Clinical Research Careers in Psychiatry. Edited by Pincus HA and Pardes H. Washington DC, American Psychiatric Press, 1986
26. Cohen DJ: Research in child psychiatry: Lines of personal, institutional and career development, in Clinical Research Careers in Psychiatry. Edited by Pincus HA and Pardes H. Washington DC, American Psychiatric Press, 1986
27. Regier DA, Burke JD: Clinical research in psychiatry: Epidemiology and services research, in Clinical Research Careers in Psychiatry. Edited by Pincus HA and Pardes H. Washington DC, American Psychiatric Press, 1986
28. Docherty JP: Clinical research in psychiatry: Psychosocial issues, in Clinical Research Careers in Psychiatry. Edited by Pincus HA and Pardes H. Washington DC, American Psychiatric Press, 1986
29. Fisher S, Bender SK: A program of research training in psychiatry: Ten-year evaluation and follow-up. Am J Psychiat 132:821-824, 1975
30. Shakow D: The education of the mental health researcher. Arch Gen Psychiat 27:15-25, 1972
31. Swisher SN: Manpower training for fundamental clinical research. Perspectives in Biology and Medicine 23 (Part 2) s62-s78, 1980
32. Levinson DJ, Darrow CN, Klein EB, et al: The Seasons of a Man's Life. New York, Knopf, 1978
33. Frazier S: personal communication, 1986

16

EDUCATIONAL MATERIALS AND TECHNOLOGY FOR THE FUTURE

Donald Fidler, M.D.

Carolyn B. Robinowitz, M.D.

The almost exponential expansion of knowledge and technology has enhanced and complicated the practice of medicine. Medical education also has been affected, not only in what is taught, but also in how it is taught.

Not too long ago, residents learned psychiatry mainly by observing. They watched faculty intervention with patients in teaching hospitals, observed inpatients, outpatients, and emergency patients, on whom they reported in supervision. Texts and journals were available for back-up, and lectures and seminars prompted discussion. Residents learned not only from faculty, but also from one another through structured and informal meetings. While didactic learning tended to be highly organized, and covered a broad range of areas of knowledge, residents' learning was dependent on the cross-section of patients they saw as well as on the availability of teaching during clinical interventions.

In psychiatry, supervision was considered to be the most important aspect of learning, providing contact with mentors and role models, opportunities to examine critically one's own clinical function and awareness, and to apply that knowledge. Supervision was, of course, an intense personal experience providing a therapeutic interaction (particularly as residents examined issues of transference and countertransference), and one of the supervisors' tasks was to differentiate this learning experience from either clinical care and consultation, or, conversely, personal psychotherapy. Supervision also was subject to the vagaries of memory and recorded notes. Residents' recall of clinical sessions often was secondary to repression of painful episodes, feelings of inadequacy, or the desire to please the supervisor. Even complicated process notes did not always replicate the actual affect or content of a therapy session.

Changes in the Future

The practice of psychiatry has undergone enormous change due to the rapid increase in knowledge and technology as well as changes in society.

Telephone intervention provides a good example of such a change. Psychiatrists and others working on "hot lines" may find themselves eliciting a history, making a diagnosis, and even conducting treatment via the telephone. Few programs teach residents about this approach, although its use by residents as well as practicing psychiatrists is increasing. This particular mode of interaction poses many problems. Residents must learn how to find out about the unseen environment of callers and assess their mood over the telephone. There is generally no immediately available supervision, nor are there guidelines for this type of work.

Video

Similarly, videotechnology is being used to a greater extent. Videotapes can provide a record of interactions with patients, as well as a library of different kinds of patients and clinical pictures. Residents must utilize a different set of clinical skills in watching a videotaped interview as contrasted with the image and feelings created in direct contacts.

While videotape is no replacement for direct patient interaction, it provides a compendium of clinical pictures including signs and symptoms, patient-physician interactions, ages, socioeconomic factors, etc. This library is always available for the needs of the student, and portions of vignettes may be used to demonstrate particular points or presentations. Other uses of videotape include demonstration of different interview styles and techniques, as well as the effect of different interventions. The Interpersonal Process Recall (IPR), developed by Norman Kagen, uses a replay of a videotaped patient interview of therapy sessions as viewed by therapist, patient, and observer/facilitator as a means of intensifying therapeutic experience and developing a higher level of communication between the patient and therapist. It also encourages greater self-awareness on the part of the therapist.

In its simplest form, the videotape may be used as a record of interventions between patient and therapist. These may provide a baseline of mood, affect, or quality of interaction over time. The videotape may assist in assessing growth of the therapist's skill. Videotapes are especially helpful in supervision, since they provide a more complete and ongoing record, without some of the problems of secondary revision that note-taking entails. Furthermore, they provide greater detail than do audiotape recordings or interviews, since the nonverbal aspects of the communication also can be displayed and analyzed. Many teachers have utilized videotaped interviews for student demonstration and discussion, both with and without the patient being present. Such a mechanism allows students to evaluate their performance and consider alternative interventions.

Teaching conferences can be videotaped. There are some hazards to this technique. It is difficult for students, often exposed to a diet of high-quality educational and entertainment television to focus on "talking heads" or a lecture. Additionally, visual materials that can aid an on-site presentation may not photograph well in a live taping. Certainly, there are some benefits to having a lecture on file, and such tapes can provide an historical record of interactions with leaders in the field. However, the best educational videotapes include carefully designed graphics and other audiovisual aids designed specifically for the medium. Such materials often are rather costly in design and execution, and involve the use of sophisticated graphics and camera techniques.

Another use of videotape involves interaction and/or simulation. Videotaped clinical vignettes may be used as a focus for discussion, emphasizing attitudes and behaviors as well as cognitively based problem-solving. H. James Lurie has developed a series of programs based on instructional videotaped vignettes consisting of brief simulated events, 30 to 90 seconds in length, designed to provoke affect, and identify and clarify attitudes and values. The videotapes also raise questions that the learners address through discussion, problem solving, and simulations, including role play. Depending upon the content, there may be a "right" or "wrong" answer, but in most instances, the identification of attitudes and clarification of values is most important. Participants also can gain a clearer understanding of how their beliefs can influence care.

Computers

There is increasing use of electronic media to replace or supplement paper and pencil. For example, written charts in many hospitals are being reduced to electronic data. The physician most be adept at using computers to read or to add information to the record, order laboratory tests, or retrieve results.

A major way that computers provide assistance is in the storage and generation of information, often too detailed to be readily available to the user. Thus, the computer can maintain data bases regarding medication, including dosage, contraindications, side effects, and even more important, interactions among drugs. Computers also can generate information about costs, e.g., comparing the price of two 50 mg tablets with that of one 100 mg tablet, attending to therapeutic benefit as well as cost-effectiveness. Computers may be used for the kind of record-keeping needed in following a clinical course of individuals or groups of patients and for engaging in research.

Thus, computers increasingly are storehouses of relevant clinical and scientific information that will no longer have to be remembered in detail by the practitioner. Data bases can be updated very rapidly. The reference system of the National Library of Medicine (Medline) is one of the best known data bases. This system, updated constantly, contains nearly all of the important medical journals covering specialties and subspecialties in English and foreign languages. Within minutes, the physician can reference the most current information on any disease, syndrome, or combination of conditions searching by key words. In many cases, a summary can be printed on the screen and downloaded for future use. Subscribers can receive copies of relevant articles mailed directly.

Specialty societies have begun to develop specialty specific data bases. Software has been created to assist psychiatrists in making DSM-III diagnoses based on clinical pictures. While these programs may not substitute for a clinical interview, they are most useful in assisting clinicians to learn problem-solving and decision-making techniques. Other software programs have been developed for pharmacological management and drug interactions. This latter is a very important area since there are increasingly greater numbers of psychotropic and other drugs, with numerous side effects and dosage schedules. This program would be particularly useful in the elderly population, since these patients may be treated concurrently for numerous psychiatric and other medical illnesses.

The computer is an excellent tool for assessment. Current paper and pencil examinations can be modified for a computer, programmed to provide answers immediately (feedback thus enhancing learning), while maintaining scores for evaluation. This approach can be used for simple, multiple choice questions, or for complex, multiply branched patient management problems. These clinical simulations can be designed to route the practitioner in certain directions; thus the end point may depend on initial or midprocess choices in an attempt to replicate clinical practice. The computer also can keep track of the number of tests ordered and their potential cost to the consumer (patient), as well as the time the diagnostic evaluation would take in real life.

Other interactive computerized learning includes videotape and/or video disc simulations of patient interactions that are portrayed on terminals through words or graphs, to a more realistic interaction between clinician and simulated patients. While some interactions demand keyboard responses, other even more sophisticated approaches will be voice responsive; that is, the clinician talks to the "patient" on screen as if the patient were real. Depending on key words programmed into the system, the "patient" responds appropriately. While this is an extremely costly approach to develop, and needs much sophisticated intervention, it is highly effective. These lifelike simulations can be used as critical incidents and interactions can be scored for safety and dangerousness, other aspects of clinical competence, as well as time use and cost-effectiveness. Their involvement of the participant in the clinical care, makes them most effective active learning tools. Furthermore, seeing immediate patient response to an intervention, tends to promote an affective response that assists the learning process.

While interactive and simulation techniques are relatively new, their development is proceeding rapidly. Decision-making on issues such as suicidality, management of violent or other difficult patients, etc., may be tested and practiced in a relatively safe setting (the simulated patient, after all, is not real) without danger to the therapist or the patient.

The computer can also be used for patient diagnostic interviews. Many patients have volunteered a preference for interacting with the computer as compared to a "real" person in such areas as history taking, interviewing, and, some have described more comfort with the computer serving as therapist, than with the physician. While these studies have not been validated scientifically, and most clinicians intuitively express concern at being replaced by a machine, no matter how sophisticated, the computer can easily be programmed to provide interventions very similar to those of some therapists. This may be a useful technique, particularly in areas where there are psychiatrist shortages. Furthermore, data can be stored and reviewed by a consulting psychiatrist who can then act as a supervisor or a second-line clinician.

Finally, computers bring clinicians located in remote areas in direct contact with experts and information in major medical centers, providing assistance in acute and ongoing care.

Telecommunications

This form of technology, although expensive to initiate, can bring together clinician experts from all over the world. Clinical conferences or other educational efforts can be broadcast simultaneously to participants in a multiplicity of settings through satellites. Technology allows for projection of charts and graphs, radiographs and photomicrographs, as well as interactive discssion among presenters, other expert consultants, and participant/trainees.

Telecommunications can add a pictorial dimension to consultation, enhancing the computer communication with a live picture of a patient interview and "face-to-face" discussion between consultant and consultee.

Conclusion

All of these technologies provide challenges and opportunities for psychiatric education and care. Their use will not compete with, but add to and complement our educational efforts in the nineties to come.

PART 3:

THE RESIDENCY PROGRAM

V. Subspecialization

There is considerable disagreement about whether to project an oversupply of psychiatrists in the 1990s. The resolution of this debate rests on the conceptualization of the roles and responsibilities of psychiatrists as opposed to other providers of mental health services. The discussion is complicated by current economic concerns demanding reduction in health care costs, citing high physician costs as one of the critical variables in its escalation. The issue is clearly more complex, and must take account of a range of factors including clinical needs, scientific and technological advances, and their impact on the nonsubstitutable activities of psychiatrists. Marketplace measures do not suffice, nor do projections of need based on the current "state-of-the-art," nor data from other countries since their philosophies and delivery systems differ substantially.

The evolution of a psychiatrist as a subspecialist appears to define a role differing from that of primary provider of mental health care. There is, however, no clear definition of the precise boundaries of subspecialization, nor is there agreement about what overlapping functions and roles will continue to be the province of the general psychiatrist and what will shift toward the subspecialist. Subspecialists, particularly child psychiatrists or geriatric psychiatrists, may provide primary care to a certain segment of the population and serve as well as consultants to other physicians (including psychiatrists) or mental health providers. Other subspecialists may function primarily as consultants (for example, forensic psychiatrists) or as primary care generalists as well as tertiary providers. The complex roles and responsibilities of today's psychiatrists as well as their multiple work settings have been well described (1), but the shape of the future remains undecided.

Conference participants deliberated these issues, but did not come to firm conclusions. Debate and discussion will, and should, continue before resolution. The arguments are delineated carefully in the papers in this section. We hope that the outcome will prove to be as we expect: closer together than they may seem at first glance. These arguments are not mutually exclusive; rather, they are complimentary. While the field appears to be moving inexorably toward increasing subspecialization, we must be cautious, yet firm; reflective, yet decisive; active, yet thoughtful. We must learn from the triumphs and errors of our medical colleagues as we forge a path to nourish our field and benefit our patients.

Carol C. Nadelson, M.D.
Carolyn B. Robinowitz, M.D.

REFERENCE

1. Langsley DG, Robinowitz CB: Psychiatric manpower: an overview. J Hosp Comm Psychiat 30:749–755, 1979

17

MANPOWER DILEMMAS

Carol C. Nadelson, M.D.

Carolyn B. Robinowitz, M.D.

Over the past decade, numerous groups have expressed concern about an undersupply of psychiatrists. These concerns led to a national conference on manpower and recruitment in psychiatry, and resulted in actions designed to increase the number of psychiatrists as well as their distribution and accessibility (1). In contrast, medical educators and manpower specialists have voiced awareness of an oversupply of physicians in general and specialists in particular (2).

In 1980, the Graduate Medical Education National Advisory Committee (GMENAC) projected that some 10,000 to 20,000 general and child psychiatrists would be needed in 1990 (2). This conclusion was based on the need for the unique services of psychiatrists as measured by the prevalence and incidence of disease, and the minimum, not necessarily optimum, non-substitutable care provided by a psychiatrist. Similar conclusions were reached by other groups which took into account the role of primary care physicians in the recognition and management of serious mental disorders, as well as the roles of nonphysician mental health providers (5). Informal reports of unfilled positions and referral practices indicate that there is still more work for psychiatrists than they are able to provide.

Health planners have used a variety of methods to estimate manpower needs. Population estimates suggest a need for about 10 psychiatrists per 100,000 population, with ranges from 6.5 to 12.5 FTE per 100,000, depending on presence of at-risk populations. In 1985, the APA estimated that there were approximately 15 psychiatrists per 100,000 population in the U.S. If these estimates are correct, and there is no redefinition of responsibilities, then the current number should be more than adequate for the 1990s. In fact, given the increasing number of medical students choosing psychiatry and reduced attrition rates due to death, illness, or retirement, it has been suggested that this need already may be met or even exceeded (4).

These numbers. however, are misleading and do not take into account the amount of service and care provided. Of the approximately 36,000 psychiatrists in the U.S., over 5,000 are residents; others are retired, in part-time practice, or engaged in research, administration, or educational activities that do not provide direct patient care (5).

Since the GMENAC report, cost considerations and other factors have had a major impact on delivery of medical care and role and function of specialists. There has been increased emphasis on managed or capitated medical care, with movement towards Health Maintenance Organizations (HMOs) and other provider-based plans that limit visits to specialists and provide incentives favoring decreased use of specialists in preference to less expensive (often nonphysician) care providers. The greater use of gatekeeper models also is a strong disincentive for specialist referral. It also is not clear what the roles will be of other "mental health professionals" whose numbers also are increasing. These allegedly less expensive therapists may deliver some of the services heretofore provided by psychiatrists. Nonetheless, these trends suggest less demand for and use of psychiatrists than GMENAC originally projected. At the same time, GMENAC did not note the impact of recent public information and education campaigns leading to more enlightened attitudes toward mental illness and psychiatric care.

Economic arguments regarding the supply of psychiatrists are generally based on marketplace models and, as such, focus on supply and demand. These often have contradictory conclusions. Marketplace theory directly links rewards paid to various types of personnel with their relative abundance. If a professional group or product is scarce, its price or reimbursement tends to rise, suggesting that lower fees for psychiatrists document an oversupply. It is clear, however, that the usual economic indicators do not necessarily apply to medical care. Most persons with an illness search for and obtain medical services whether or not they have the resources to pay for care. Treatment tends to be dispensed first, and payment comes later. Catastrophic or major chronic illnesses produce treatment needs and expenses beyond the capacities of most persons to pay. Furthermore, reimbursement seems less to be related to scarcity of resources and more to the degree of high technology and complex procedures, such that the high-risk or "high-tech" care such as open heart surgery provides a higher professional fee. Thus, although there is no shortage of surgeons, and in fact, an estimated oversupply exists, surgeons receive high fees for technical procedures. The family physician or psychiatrist who provides more time and labor-intensive but "low-tech" care, is reimbursed at a significantly lower rate.

Other economists state that the numbers of physicians should be increased, expecting fees charged to be lowered in the face of increased competition. Still a third group has noted that since each physician generates a certain amount of medical costs regardless of how many physicians there are, the supply of physicians should be limited to minimize cost (6).

Other arguments relating to manpower needs are concerned more with distribution than with actual numbers. Yet, there must be a sufficient critical mass to effect changes in distribution patterns. Yager and Borus, supporting the concept of oversupply, make the assumption we should discontinue residencies mainly attracting Foreign Medical Graduates (FMGs) who receive little or poor training and work mainly to provide services in large state facilities (7). Their proposal for hiring fully trained psychiatrists to provide this care does not address the shortage of care givers in such settings, and documents the undersupply as well as the maldistribution.

Arguments regarding supply also must consider the roles and responsibilities of psychiatrists and what functions are substitutable, that is, can be provided by nonpsychiatrists. There is no question that there is already an existing, large, unmet need for mental health services. Conservative estimates place 15 percent of the population and more than 32 million people in need of mental health services in any given year. Who should provide their care?

If psychiatrists are responsible for primary health care, they will have a critical role in triage, treatment planning, as well as service delivery, but estimates of need will be higher. If, on the other hand, the psychiatrist is conceptualized primarily as a consultant to nonphysician mental health professionals or other physicians, thus providing indirect care, then the number of psychiatrists needed will be far fewer.

The definition of a psychiatrist as a practitioner with increasing interest, knowlege, and skill as a subspecialist appears to differ from the role of primary provider of mental health care. Such a definition, however, does not address the actual roles, functions, or boundaries of subspecialty practice, and confuses subspecialization with consultation. Many subspecialists, particularly child and adolescent psychiatrists or geriatric psychiatrists, continue to provide direct primary care not only to their targeted subspecialty patient populations, but also to other psychiatric patients in addition to their consultative roles with other physicians (including psychiatrists), mental health or social service providers. Furthermore, an increase in the knowledge base and options for care available may lead to greater consumer demand for services, and thus, greater manpower needs. Increased consultation to and education of other providers also can lead to increased diagnosis and referrals for care.

Measuring the need for health care and associated manpower is problematic. We continue to deal with human variability and an ill-defined set of "products," provided by a variety of practitioners with a variety of skills and knowledge. The question of role and responsibility must be addressed before determination of either need or demand can be made.

Thus, arguments can be made from either perspective oversupply or undersupply. At this time, there are no conclusive data to settle the question. It is critical, however, to make decisions about what level of evaluation, diagnosis, and treatment can be performed by other providers; what training they must have to function effectively to deliver high-quality mental health care; as well as who shall assume responsibility for their training and performance evaluation.

Finally, a combination of availability of care, economics, education of patient population, and sociopolitical issues will interact with epidemiologic factors, treatment methodologies, practitioner skills, and practice patterns to determine the number and type of care givers needed and utilized. Nonetheless, in the nineties and thereafter, we must recruit the best U.S. medical students to enter the field, to maintain the vitality of the profession and continually to improve the quality of care we can provide.

References

1. Robinowitz CB, Taintor Z: A national conference on recruitment into psychiatry: conference recommendations. J Med Ed 5:168-178, 1981

2. Office of Graduate Medical Eduation, Health Resources Administration: Report of the Graduate Medical Education National Advisory Committee. Washington DC, DHHS Pub. No. HRA 81-652, 1980
3. Koran LM: Psychiatric manpower ratios: A beguiling numbers game. Arch Gen Psychiat 36:1409-1415, 1979
4. Yager J, Borus J: Are we training too many psychiatrists? Am J Psychiat (in Press)
5. American Psychiatric Association: 1983 Census of Members, unpublished data
6. Robinowitz CB: Is there a shortage of psychiatrists? A psychiatrist's response. Comm Ment Hlth 19:54-58, 1983
7. Yager J, Borus J: Are we training too many psychiatrists? Am J Psychiat (in Press)

18

THE FUTURE PSYCHIATRIST AS SUBSPECIALIST: THERE IS NO ALTERNATIVE

Joel Yager, M.D.

Donald G. Langsley, M.D.

Roger Peele, M.D.

F. Patrick McKegney, M.D.

Paul Fink, M.D.

During the 1930s, psychiatry officially became a medical specialty. The American Board of Psychiatry and Neurology (ABPN) was established and joined the American Board of Medical Specialties (ABMS) (1). Psychiatry now faces another evolutionary leap. The generalist psychiatrist, as the general medical practitioner of generations ago, will yield to the subspecialist psychiatrist.

This change will not necessarily lead to the development of subspecialist psychiatrists as narrowly focused practitioners, wearing blinders to clinical issues beyond their subspecialty. Rather, they will become highly skilled in specific areas, and this expertise will be built upon a firm grounding in general psychiatry. They will focus primarily on the biological syndromes of psychiatry, work with patients with psychiatric responses to medical illnesses, and act as consultants to other health care providers and/or organizations.

For many psychiatrists who derive their deepest professional satisfaction from the practice of general psychiatry, the spectre of subspecialization is not greeted with enthusiasm. These psychiatrists are loathe to cede the treatment of a variety of patients over time, utilizing many different kinds of interventions and treatment modalities. They are concerned that clinical practice, as it now exists, might disappear forever.

Such fears are ill-founded. Similar gratifications are available within subspecialty practice. Studies have demonstrated that many medical subspecialists continue to practice primary care medicine as well as their subspecialty (2). Practitioners of emerging psychiatric subspecialties are not necessarily exclusively wedded to subspecialty practice; they also engage in a significant amount of general psychiatry, and most likely will continue to do so.

This paper describes the internal and external forces that are leading inexorably toward subspecialty training and practice; suggesting that psychiatrists actively engage in shaping that future, rather than allowing time to simply take its toll. If grounded in firm direction from the profession itself, this new course for our specialty should be welcomed.

Defining Basic Psychiatric Skills

Langsley and Hollender (3) have described the skills required of a psychiatric specialist, based upon a wide range of psychiatrists' opinions. The core skills include the ability to diagnose psychiatric disorders and to provide individual psychodynamic psychotherapy and phamacological therapy. Beyond these skills, there is little agreement about those areas of knowledge and training that should be maintained as part of the core residency curriculum and those that are more suited for inclusion in a subspecialty curriculum.

Some of the skills cited by Langsley and Hollender include those that also are shared with nonpsychiatric physicians and non-physician mental health professionals. The list of non-substitutable psychiatric skills includes: comprehensive physical and mental assessment and diagnosis of patients with mental illness, overall treatment planning and management of such patients, treatment of patients whose conditions require concurrent medication and psychotherapy, supervision and consultation with primary care physicians and other mental health clinicians in complicated cases, application of ECT and other somatic treatments, and the practice of forensic psychiatry. These skills will remain the province of psychiatrists because only this profession primarily works with the biological syndromes of psychiatry: in diagnosis, distinguishing the biological, psychological and social contributors to psychiatric disorders; in treatment planning, coordinating biological, psychological and social interventions; and in treatment follow-up, monitoring treatment efficacy across all spheres of intervention. In addition to attention to the biopsychosocial arts and sciences of psychiatry, basic training in general psychiatry (10) includes additional emphasis on scientific thinking, through critical analysis of the literature and participation in research.

In other areas, there is relatively little to differentiate psychiatrists from other physicians and/or nonphysician mental health professionals. The practice of psychotherapy, central to the professional identity and activities of most psychiatrists, no longer distinguishes psychiatrists from other practitioners. Indeed, while the knowledge, attitudes, and skills acquired by training in individual psychotherapy as well as other types of psychotherapy provide an essential perspective for all psychiatrists, the future psychiatrists will not practice utilizing only psychotherapy skills. Many other mental health disciplines are prepared to conduct psychotherapy with many of the same patient populations seen by psychiatrists. The data suggest that these practitioners may be able to do so with equal capacity.

Similarly, in psychopharmacology, where psychiatrists should certainly claim unique expertise, the primary care specialties have recommended that family medicine and internal medicine specialists gain familiarity and competence with at least minor tranquilizers and tricyclic anti-depressants (7). At this time, the use of monamine oxidase inhibitors, neuroleptics, lithium, and a few other major pharmacologic agents continues to remain with psychiatrists, but it is hard to justify psychiatry's identity based upon this relatively small list.

Although the potential role of psychiatry as a primary care specialty has been advocated (4), the consensus of opinion on the part of physicians is that it is more appropriate that general physicians provide primary care for psychiatric patients (5) and that psychiatrists function as specialists rather than primary care givers. Indeed, the evidence indicates that when psychiatrists are faced with difficult or ambiguous medical decisions, despite their level of training or practice, they are inclined to call for specialist consultation rather than to take responsibility for diagnosing the patient's medical problems on their own (6). Thus, as psychiatrists specialize, their practices will increasingly focus on tertiary, highly circumscribed spheres of care, built upon a strong biopsychosocial knowledge base.

Forces Within the Profession Supporting Subspecialization

Over the past 25 years, subspecialization in all fields of medicine has moved inexorably ahead, motivated principally by the search for quality medical care. Although there has been some concern about fragmentation of patient care, the explosion of medical science and technology has made it virtually impossible for physicians to maintain awareness of the entire field, much less of their own specialty, or subspecialty areas.

Psychiatrists today often restrict their practice, even without formal subspecialty credentials. Psychiatric subspecialty areas have generally emerged from specific areas of expertise or population groups (e.g., forensic, child, adolescent, geriatric), specific disorders (e.g., schizophrenia, affective disorders, substance abuse), specific techniques (e.g., psychopharmacology, ECT), or other domains in which psychiatrists work (e.g., family therapy or administrative psychiatry). With an increase in knowledge and technology, we can expect other subdivisions and subspecialty interests to evolve.

Subspecialties develop and are recognized when a body of scientific knowledge and skill becomes distinguishable; when a group of physicians concentrate their practice in that area; when specialty journals or texts are published; when national societies, focused on that area of expertise, develop; and when medical schools or hospitals devote courses, divisions, training time, and personnel to that clinical area.

The American Board of Medical Specialties (ABMS) now recognizes over 80 specialist and subspecialist credentials. Internal medicine has twelve subspecialties; pediatrics has eight; obstetrics and gynecology has four; pathology has nine. Currently, psychiatry has only one ABMS recognized, credentialed subspecialty, child psychiatry. There are, however, a number of emerging subspecialties. Possible candidates for ABMS recognition and American Board of Psychiatry and Neurology (ABPN) certification are detailed in Appendix A.

Subspecialization is also presaged by the publication of subspecialty journals such as the Journal of Clinical Psychopharmacology, the Journal of Affective Disorders, the International Journal of Eating Disorders, among others. Similarly, movement in the profession and the demands for professionals with special skills has led to the emergence of a variety of psychiatric post-graduate fellowship programs, even in the absence of certifying boards. In many urban areas and academic centers, cross referral among subspecialists within psychiatry is now commonplace. A psychiatrist with one area of interest is more inclined to refer complicated or difficult patients, or patients whose problems are outside the psychiatrist's area to others working more intensively with those populations.

Forces Outside the Profession Supporting Subspecialization

Trends in contemporary medical practice and economics, e.g., increased numbers of prepaid group plans, increased utilization of "alternative" care providers, and questions about service efficacy, may stimulate subspecialization in psychiatry. The "HMO-ization" of American medicine (8, 9) will have an effect upon future psychiatric practice. Many of these prepaid systems utilize a gatekeeper model for referral whereby patients are seen by specialists only upon referral from primary care physicians or other "gatekeepers." Today, many plans, for example Medicaid in Arizona and the UCLA "HealthNet" plan, incorporate strong disincentives for primary care providers to refer to specialists. The fees for specialist care come out of a financial "pot" controlled by the primary care providers. For purely economic reasons, visits to specialists and the conditions under which specialists can be seen, are limited. Only more complicated or resistant patients are referred to psychiatrists under this system.

At the same time, the huge for-profit corporations that are increasingly controlling medical care are following the path already set by community mental health centers (8, 9). These corporations will define the tasks to be performed by various mental health providers and specify the numbers of each type needed. They will demand scientific data assessing the effectiveness of psychiatric interventions, comparing the outcome to that of other types of treatment by nonphysician mental health professionals (9). If treatment-related positive changes in patient functioning can be demonstrated, and if psychiatrists can be shown to be more effective and efficient providers of care than others, psychiatrists will have a role in primary treatment of the mentally ill in the future. Otherwise, psychiatrists will serve predominantly as consultants to other, less expensive "generic therapists," such as psychologists, social workers and psychiatric nurses, who are entering the field at far more rapid rates (10, 11).

The experience in Great Britain, where the gatekeeper model has been in place for some years, provides additional evidence that in the future, psychiatrists are likely to be more involved as consultants, teachers, and researchers than in primary care (12). To some extent, British psychiatrists may already be living our future, since their role has been restructured in response to economic constraints.

Psychiatry Should Direct the Future of Subspecialization

Psychiatry will be ill served if the inevitable trend toward subspecialization is allowed to evolve spontaneously. Without direction from the profession, psychiatry can become a patchwork, incomprehensible to prospective patients, to the public, and, eventually, even to professionals. Overlapping subspecialties will fight for patients; patients will not know who should serve them; public-policy makers will not know who speaks to what problem; professionals will not know who is responsible for which patient.

In order to guide this trend, psychiatric leaders should adopt a specific conceptual framework to organize subspecialization along parameters that will minimize confusion and conflict. There are at least five groupings of subspecialization:

- Functional subspecialization: administrative, clinical, consultation-liaison, forensic, occupational, preventive/public health, research, teaching, etc.
- Employer subspecialization: community mental health center, correctional institution, government, general hospital, academic, HMO, military, public sector, private hospital, private office, etc.
- Treatment site subspecialization: office (outpatient, clinic, ambulatory care), day treatment, inpatient.
- Knowledge/treatment/procedure subspecialization: ECT, milieu therapy, psychopharmacology, psychotherapy (individual including psychoanalysis, behavioral psychotherapy; group; family; etc.), rehabilitation, and others.
- Patient subspecialization: age (child, geriatric), ethnic or racial, gender, nonpsychiatric handicapped (e.g., specialist in blind or deaf), psychiatric disorder (e.g., specialist in affective disorders, eating disorders, etc.).

Of these groupings, the last, patient subspecialization, seems to meet the needs of the patients and public policy makers better than the others. While no model will abolish intraprofessional or interprofessional conflicts altogether, subspecialization by age of the patient and by diagnosis narrows the conflict most substantially. Under this model questions about one's share of the marketplace are less a function of "winning out" over other subspecialists than they are if subspecialization is based on procedure, treatment site or employer.

If we accept this model of subspecialization, the psychiatrist of the future should be a highly skilled diagnostician, subspecializing in a major subgroup of patients, defined by age and/or by diagnosis. Paralleling the model of internal medicine subspecialties, future psychiatrists should be able to evaluate any patient who comes to them, retaining treatment responsibility for those in their subspecialty. Clearly, this model also suggests training goals for the future.

Implications for Education and Training

The evolution of psychiatry into a series of subspecialties with a core of general psychiatric knowledge has important implications for training and will provide an incentive for focusing on increasing the quality of psychiatric education, and on certifying the competence of our graduates. Additional education and training will be rigorously assessed (12).

Even programs that predominantly train general psychiatrists should be expected to have faculty expert in major subspecialty areas. Those residency programs that do not include subspecialist faculty foster the illusion that there is not much to know, or that knowledge beyond the core curriculum is irrelevant to the profession. The Residency Review Committee for Psychiatry (RRC) should ascertain that program faculty is qualified to provide subspecialist training in major areas such as child psychiatry, psychopharmacology, psychodynamics, geriatrics, among others. Adoption of specific requirements by the RRC would parallel training procedures already mandated in internal medicine and pediatrics where the resident is taught by both generalists and subspecialists. Training requirements in those fields specify that faculty must include subspecialists, and PGY-3 residents in those fields spend nearly half of their time in subspecialty rotations. Similarly, psychiatry should provide a continuum of subspecialty rotations and tracks during residency and into post-graduate subspeciality fellowships.

To increase the quality of those training to become psychiatric specialists, a certification process should be set in place at the end of training (13). In the future, all psychiatric residents should be certified before they are considered psychiatrists. Those training in subspecialties should be fully trained to evaluate any psychiatrically ill patient and, in addition, to treat those within a major age and/or diagnostic subspecialty grouping.

Conclusion

Psychiatry inevitably will evolve into a discipline with multiple subspecialties. We must structure this evolution to ensure that such developments are beneficial, resulting in increased rather than decreased vitality and productivity. This will require increased quality control in our recruitment, training, and certification processes, leading to increased accountability of the profession. The basic professional satisfactions available in the practice of general psychiatry will not disappear. Rather, superimposed on the strengths of such general preparation, the special skills and expertise of the subspecialist will enable psychiatry to flourish.

References

1. Rudy LH: American Board of Psychiatry and Neurology in Comprehensive Textbook of Psychiatry, IV. Edited by Kaplan HI, Sadock BJ. Baltimore MD, Williams and Wilkins, 1985
2. Aiken LH, Lewis CE, Craig J, et al: The contribution of specialists to the delivery of primary care: A new perspective. NEJM 300:1363-1370, 1979
3. Langsley D, Hollender M: The definition of a psychiatrist. Am J Psychiat 139:81-85, 1982
4. Fink PJ, Oken D: The role of psychiatry as a primary care specialty. Arch Gen Psychiat 33:998-1003, 1976
5. Hankin J, Oktay JS: Mental disorders and primary medical care: An analytic review of the literature. DHEW Publication No. (ADM) 78-661. Washington DC, US Government Printing Office, 1979
6. Yager J, Linn LS, Leake B, et al: Initial clinical judgments by internists, family physicians and psychiatrists in response to patient vignettes. II. Ordering laboratory tests, consultation and treatments. Gen Hosp Psychiat, in press, 1986
7. American Psychiatric Association: Psychiatric Education and the Primary Care Physician: Task Force Report 2. Washington DC, American Psychiatric Association, 1970
8. Tarlov AR: The increasing supply of physicians, the changing structure of the health-service system and the future practice of medicine. NEJM 308:1235-1244, 1983
9. Geyman JP: Future medical practice in the United States: A choice of scenarios. JAMA 245:1140-1144, 1981
10. Jenkins J, Turk V: Mental health manpower, in Mental Health, United States 1983. Edited by Taube CA, Barrett SA. DHHS

Pub No. (ADM) 83-1275. Rockville MD, National Institute of Mental Health, 1983
11. Karls JM: Mental health manpower production study No. 1: Selected preliminary findings. Sacramento CA, California State Department of Mental Health, 1984
12. Crisp AH, Hemsi LK, Paykel ES, et al: A future pattern of psychiatric service and its educational implications: Some suggestions. J Med Ed 18:110-116, 1984
13. Borus JF, Yager J: Ongoing evaluation in psychiatry: The first step toward quality. Am J Psychiat, accepted for publication, 1986

APPENDIX A

EMERGING SUBSPECIALTIES IN PSYCHIATRY

A number of fields are emerging as psychiatric subspecialties, with requisite training, recognition and credentialing processes either in place or under consideration. Undoubtedly, with additional knowledge, others will appear.

CHILD PSYCHIATRY. Already a recognized subspecialty, child psychiatry is attempting to increase its academic and scientific base, and to recruit needed practitioners.

GERIATRIC PSYCHIATRY. This field has been recognized as a subspecialty area by internal and family medicine as well as psychiatry. Increasing service needs are demanding increased numbers of specialists. Its scientific base is growing and numerous post-graduate fellowship positions already exist.

PSYCHOANALYSIS. A subspecialty neither limited to psychiatrists nor recognized within medicine, psychoanalysis increasingly has opened is educational programs to nonphysicians, setting up credentialing processes outside psychiatry. While psychoanalytic programs which focus on physicians could become more closely allied with psychiatry and identified as a subspecialty, it would be difficult to demonstrate how training or expertise in this area differs from that of nonphysician psychoanalysts.

FORENSIC PSYCHIATRY. This field has both recognized fellowships and a certification process, albeit outside the ABMS/ABPN. It could become part of mainstream psychiatric credentialing through the ABPN.

CONSULTATION-LIAISON PSYCHIATRY. Fellowship training and national societies already exist. Whether subspecialization is warranted is not yet clear.

CLINICAL PSYCHOPHARMACOLOGY. Fellowship training, national societies, journals, and the potential for development as a recognized subspecialty are all in evidence. Such subspecialists already function as consultants on difficult cases for many general psychiatrists, for nonpsychiatric physicians, and for mental health workers.

ADMINISTRATIVE PSYCHIATRY. The American Psychiatric Association, but not the ABPN, has already recognized and certified psychiatrists in administrative psychiatry. There are not yet many training programs, but the field has national societies and a national interest.

19

THE FUTURE ROLE OF PSYCHIATRISTS

Melvin Sabshin, M.D.

This paper addresses the statement developed for debate on the future role of psychiatrists:

> *The psychiatrist of the nineties will not practice as a psychiatric generalist utilizing psychotherapy skills, but will primarily practice as a subspecialist psychiatric physician working with the biological syndromes of psychiatry, patients with a psychiatric response to medical illness, and as consultants to other health care providers and/or organizations.*

The nihilists, including some anti-psychiatrists, believe that mental health services should be demedicalized and that there is no medical role. Another group states that medicine is irrelevant and criticizes, for example, the need for formal diagnosis and epidemiology. This group rejects medical nosology for being reductionistic and longs for the return of a halcyon period when dynamic psychothrerapy had much more power in American psychiatry. Another group believes that psychiatry will be subsumed as a part of neurology in the future, and that there is no special need for education in psychotherapy.

The statement that the psychiatrist of the 1990s will not utilize psychotherapy in practice implies that a subspecialist does essentially everything in psychiatry, except the practice of psychotherapy. Thus, subspecialization is defined by exclusion, and the addition of psychotherapy is what defines the generalist. Actuarial data support the assertion that most psychiatrists age 50 and under will continue to practice into the next century. As such, they will not give up their utilization of psychotherapy as a main or adjunct treatment for many patients with mental disorders, including those with such biological syndromes as manic depressive disorder, and patients with psychiatric problems resulting from other medical illnesses. By far the most common form of current treatment practice involves a combination of psychotherapy and psychopharmacotherapy. This pattern will surely continue. Hopefully, the psychiatrist of the nineties (and thereafter) will avoid the reductionism inherent in polarizing either biological treatment or psychotherapy, but will use a mixture of the two as is appropriate. Psychiatrists work with patients rather than with biological syndromes, psychotherapy is included as an integral part of that work.

In addition, referring patients to other health care providers for the psychotherapy "portion" of treatment is inefficient and ineffective, and a poor treatment model. Issues of compliance, the impact and effect of medication, including the relation of medication to a patient's psychological functioning and self-esteem and/or the brief need for medication at times of crisis or exacerbation should be integrated into a treatment approach rather than delegated to a psychopharmacologic specialist. While psychiatrists can serve as consultants in when medication is needed in addition to ongoing psychotherapy, these instances should be integrated into patient care.

Arguments against the continued use of psychotherapy by psychiatrists have hinged on cost effectiveness as well as greater acceptability of nonpsychiatrists as psychotherapists; both premises are fallacious. Psychiatrists do not necessarily cost more, particularly if they provide integrative functions. While some argue that there is greater acceptability of psychotherapy provided by nonpsychiatrist physicians or other mental health practitioners since it is seen as less stigmatizing, there are not good data to support that premise. Further, the duplicative approach is less efficient and more expensive. The complex monitoring needed offsets the potential benefits.

Some psychiatrists will continue to practice psychoanalysis and long-term psychotherapy. There also will be a general tendency toward briefer and more focused psychotherapies, behavior therapies, group and family approaches. As such, the psychiatrist should have a diverse clinical armamentarium. In the nineties, there will be a clearer explication of the most appropriate choice of therapies for specific patients with defined disorders.

In working with patients with a "psychiatric response to medical illness," psychotherapy is often most appropriate. While some responses lend themselves to psychopharmacologic intervention, most patients require integrated treatment. In many instances, psychopharmacologic agents may even be contraindicated. In any event, psychotherapy can be used to help patients to come to terms with severe, chronic, or disfiguring illnesses, and as an adjunct to other medical treatment aimed directly at the nonpsychiatric disorder.

Moreover, it should be obvious that psychiatrists cannot be consultants to other providers of psychotherapy without continuing to practice psychotherapy and being knowledgeable in the implications, indications, as well as the special aspects of this treatment.

The affirmative statement of this debate implies a significant degree of biological reductionism. If it becomes reality, it may help to achieve the deepest aspirations of those who have been predicting the demise of the field. Psychiatric treatment will be depersonalized, mechanized, and trivialized, if not deadly dull. The options for practice will be limited if the psychosocial components are removed from the list of psychiatrists' skills.

The alternative to reductionism is not limited to caring humanistic practices; rather, all treatment should be grounded in empiricism and scientific principles. Further, a diagnostic and integrative capacity will be among the core and unique skills of the psychiatrist in the 1990s, differentiating psychiatrists from other medical specialists and mental health care providers. Understanding psychotherapy and psychodynamic psychological and behavioral functions will contribute to these diagnostic skills.

What is unique about psychiatry is its integrative, empirically based and theoretically sound spanning of psychosocial and biological approaches. Most important is the capacity to formulate a differential diagnosis, to make a rational choice of treatment, and to carry out the treatment, making the necessary adjustments and follow-up. Thus, the skills of the psychiatrist in the nineties will be more than the pooling of services of a psychologist and neurologist. The generalist will most often use a mixture of combined techniques, and will be able to titrate each, or move from one to the other with a diverse age and sex-stratified sample of patients.

This centrality of diagnosis, not by a checklist, but with treatment planning and treatment follow-up, provides a comprehensive breadth of skills and functions as implicit definitions of a psychiatrist and generalist. The definition of a consultant includes interpersonal skills. The failure to learn or use those skills limits breadth of function and understanding, and ultimately weakens the capacity to consult or to recommend the appropriate treatment.

Subspecialization

Subspecialization, as has been stated, can be conceptualized by age (infant, child, adolescent, geriatric); by special forms of intervention or system-oriented specialists (forensic); by depth of experience and concentration (psychophamacology or psychoanalysis); by disease entity (substance abuse, eating disorders), etc. Obviously, subspecialization will continue, because as the knowledge base of the field has expanded, so has interest in subspecialization. Psychiatrists have emulated other physicians in focusing or limiting their practices, and they have emphasized one or more areas of special knowledge or expertise, or approaches. This emphasis has been supported by hospitals which express interest in determining whether physician staff members have certain abilities by virtue of training or experience. These hospitals are beginning to award privileges not only by specialty, but by demonstrated knowledge or skills. As an example, in some hospitals, psychiatrists must demonstrate expertise in procedures such as ECT before receiving privileges to perform them.

Competitive interests also have prompted subspecialty focus. Increasing numbers of clinics or facilities are specializing in disorders (e.g., addictions, eating disorders, mood disorders) or special populations (for example, for the elderly, children and youth, dual diagnosis of physically ill patients). Such facilities have not only provided a site for care with resources and expertise located in a single site, but they have provided greater opportunities for scientific study of their patients, as well as competition in the marketplace.

Other specialties have focused on developing subspecialty training certification and practice (with the specialty boards providing certificates of added or special qualifications), requiring one, two, or even three years of post-residency training. The intense growth in internal medicine corresponds with the growth of its subspecialty areas in the past two decades. Just as the specialty of internal medicine as been weakened in part by the immense growth of subspecialty practice, it is feared that the unified force now representing psychiatry as a whole could be modified to a group of small and sometimes competing subspecialty organizations and approaches. Indeed, the generalist, too, becomes a specialist. Psychiatry has a great need to convey to decision-makers and the general public that it has become organized on an empirical and clinical scientific base. Will the development of multiple subspecialties weaken this perception, particularly with the emergence of less scientifically based subspecialties? What will be the effect on the field's drive toward unification?

These issues are complex and somewhat contradictory. Many academicians believe the way to promote advancement and growth in scientific knowledge in academic psychiatry is to subspecialize. Thus, many academic departments have formed subspecialty or quasi-subspecialty divisions with distinct clinical service tracks, fellowship programs, research efforts, and didactic responsibilities. Congruent with this increase in knowledge, there has been a significant growth of formal and informal training experiences available in subspecialty areas. Some training is offered as elective opportunities during the residency, but increasingly more is provided through a full-time or part-time post-residency experience. Each year, a larger number of psychiatry residents opt for a fifth or sixth post-graduate year to pursue an area in greater depth.

While the formation of subspecialty fellowship programs might lead to less subspecialty teaching in the general residency, experience in internal medicine has demonstrated that the growth of the subspecialty fellowships parallel stronger content in general internal medicine training programs. Nonetheless, those who are interested in geriatric or forensic psychiatry might be forced to take a fellowship to obtain sufficient training exposure. There is no doubt about whether there will be sufficient funding to develop these specialized fellowship training programs at a time when funding for graduate medical education, and, for that matter, medical care, increasingly has been limited.

Questions have been raised about the economic impact of subspecialization. Currently, there are few financial incentives to be board certified, and certification is not required for specialty practice. Will the emergence of a plethora of subspecialty areas have an adverse effect on those who choose to practice as generalists? What effect will it have on the psychiatrists who have chosen to limit or focus their practice to one or more specialty areas, but who have had clinical experience, rather than formal training or certification to support their expertise? Furthermore, what is the increased potential for malpractice litigation, and how will we determine the standard of care for generalists working in a specialty area such as geriatrics, or specialists who also provide generalist care? Will the growth of subspecialty areas limit care by the generalist psychiatrists? Are there enough specialists to handle the needs? Most general psychiatrists, for example, provide care for some portion of the elderly population. Would growth of subspecialties deny care to some of these elderly persons, or deny general psychiatrists the opportunity to provide such care? How would this subspecialization affect the cost of care?

Clearly, subspecialists will be needed, and they are being developed. We must integrate their contributions with those of the generalist, increasing the knowledge base of both. Psychiatry is in a growth phase in terms of the knowledge and scientific information available. A major task of the nineties will be the integration of the knowledge and skills, both current and projected, and the avoidance of reductionism or premature closure.

PART 3:

THE RESIDENCY PROGRAM

VI. Evaluation

Examinations serve multiple purposes. It is essential that these not be merged or blended, and that the specific goals of an examination be identified and made explicit to both evaluator and test-taker. Individual certification and program assessment are different tasks, and the evaluations to achieve these goals should be developed separately under the appropriate organizational auspices. The methodology of the examination, and the areas examined should be specific to the function for which the examination is designed.

The first two papers set forth differing views of the role of examinations in psychiatric residency training. Gardner suggests that examinations fail to test necessary cognitive skills and that they serve as artificial end-point measures, not necessarily reflective of either resident knowledge or, even more important, issues of ethics and critical thinking. He poses an alternative system of ongoing "feedback loops" during residency that provides ongoing assessment of resident knowledge and direction for further education. Shader, acknowledging that current assessment techniques fall short of the mark, suggests a mechanism whereby appropriate assessment through examination can be achieved to the benefit of both resident trainee and training program.

The final paper in this section by Tasman and Rieder sets forth one type of evaluation mechanism—the critical incident evaluation simulation technique—as a means of either providing the "feedback loop" suggested by Gardner or of evaluating resident competence at the termination of training, as suggested by Shader. The authors detail the development, structure, and conduct of this technique for use by resident training faculty.

Stefan Stein, M.D.

20

A COGNITIVE EXAMINATION FOR RESIDENCY GRADUATION IS NOT NECESSARY

Russell Gardner, Jr., M.D.

Psychiatric training programs are under increasing pressure to guarantee that their graduates meet standards of high quality. More than 90 percent of residency training programs assess resident knowledge through the Psychiatry Residency In-Training Examination (PRITE). Some educators have suggested that residents should be required to pass a cognitive test such as the PRITE in order to graduate.

Passing a cognitive examination should not be the only criterion for graduation, since such exams are generally inadequate to skills assessment. Sole reliance on such a process would short-circuit the development of difficult and complex but clearly more adequate faculty involvement in the process of assessment and evaluation. Evaluation practices should be closely intertwined with the educational process, beginning early in training and continuing throughout residency. Evaluation should not be left to an anxiety-producing "final examination."

This paper proposes means of achieving high quality residents without requiring a cognitive examination. It seeks to balance the public need for better quality control against the equally compelling need to link education and evaluation throughout the course of a residency, within the scope of current educational evaluation techniques.

The Need for Appropriate Evaluation

Psychiatrists work not only with patients, but with employers, insurance carriers, courts, and the public. All of these groups demand assurance of the competence of the psychiatrist. Those charged with training responsibility must maintain appropriate standards. These should be determined by criteria more exacting than a resident's demonstration of test-taking skills and abilities.

More critical to determining a psychiatrist's competence are such questions as: what is the psychiatrist's ability to gather information critical to making diagnostic assessments and treatment determinations, and to apply that knowledge? Can the psychiatrist appropriately deploy, and then evaluate the efficacy of chosen treatments? What is the quality of the resident's judgment and ethics? These questions demand evaluation of qualities that can only be suggested by the results of cognitive examinations.

Problems with Existing Methods

Currently, psychiatric certification procedures are more focused and demanding than are the requirements for graduation from a residency training program. During the residency, the PRITE exam is available as a tool with which residents are able to assess their knowledge base, compared with their peers, at particular points in the program. Residents not only learn what their performance is on a standardized test, but also receive a list of correct answers and references for those answers. PRITE does not assess either resident competence or program quality. It does help prepare the resident for later certification procedures, through an assessment of content knowledge.

The ABPN Part One written examination provides an assessment independent of the residency program. Like other cognitive examinations, it is insensitive to interpersonal variables. The ABPN Part Two examination evaluates interviewing skills and performance through observation by a panel of examiners. This exam measures capacity to gather and assess patient information and demonstrate problem-solving skills. Attitudes and interpersonal skills may be demonstrated during this assessment, but there are limits to the exam procedure itself. Evaluation in this setting becomes a criterion for certification.

Unfortunately, this kind of oral examination is vulnerable to error, in part because of the extraordinary anxiety generating pressure involved in the process. Thus, what is being examined may not be clinical competence, but the maintenance of clinical ability in a particularly stressful situation. Two one-hour oral examinations are inadequate to determine a psychiatrist's professional behavior, his or her competence, ethical judgment, and professional demeanor. While the credentialing process is the initial phase of certification, and it provides some assurance that the candidate has completed a residency and demonstrated requisite knowledge, there are variations in levels required for "graduation." Residency training directors do not have to attest to the level of a candidate's skills and competence. Moreover, because physicians need not become board certified to practice psychiatry, many graduates do not even enter the certification process.

Thus, there is difficulty assessing the quality of residents during training, and we have no external review of the quality of those psychiatrists who opt not to enter the ABPN certifying process. Recently, two proposals have been made. One is to assign a fourth year gatekeeping responsibility to the PRITE exam; the other is to move the ABPN exam into the final residency year. Both could have deleterious effects upon our residency programs and do not serve the purposes for which the two examinations were initially developed. PRITE would lose its value as an ongoing evaluative and educational tool; the ABPN Part One would no longer have a post-residency credentialing and certifying mechanism. Moreover, each would serve only as one-time gatekeeping examinations—high anxiety-ridden experiences that reflect competence only dubiously, but allow a simple "out" for the discipline.

Ideal Evaluation Processes

Delayed feedback, such as that provided by an end-of-training examination, is a poor method for correcting behavior. The trainee who fails so late in the training process, may be justifiably upset. Unfortunately, this evaluative process does not recognize the link between education and evaluation which should be established throughout the training. Evaluation should occur at all points in resident education and should have feedback loops to remediate weaknesses. One kind of short-term feedback loop is provided by the critical incident technique which provides simulations of diagnosis and assessment situations. The resident's performance is then graded by the supervisor against pre-established criteria. Results then influence further educational programs. Such a procedure should be part of the everyday experience of the resident.

Residency programs should have mechanisms for recording the content of those evaluations. This systematic documentation would be a benefit to residents by aiding in their future credentialing and professional growth. It also would stimulate resident professional growth and educational development.

Conclusion

The idea of using PRITE or any other cognitive examination as a rite of passage from residency to psychiatric practice should be discarded. PRITE should be maintained as an educational tool during residency. A system of linkages between education and evaluation should extend throughout graduate education. Residency programs should develop methods of extensive easy-to-use documentation of resident performance. At the same time, the field should develop mechanisms other than paper and pencil tests to evaluate trainees' clinical skills and behavior. Simulations such as critical incidents can serve this function.

21

THE VALUE OF AN IN-SERVICE EXAMINATION IN PSYCHIATRY

Richard I. Shader, M.D.

Psychiatric training programs are diverse in orientation, varying in depth and breadth of faculty, curricular format, size of peer group, and type of training setting. The use of standardized, mandatory, in-service examinations would ensure that graduates of such diverse programs have mastered a comparable body of knowledge and have acquired psychiatric skills and proficiency. Such examinations also may help residency programs assess their curricular strengths and weaknesses, promoting corrective adjustments in the programs themselves. Just as we require graduates of foreign medical schools to demonstrate individual proficiency through examination, we should require our residents to pass an examination as a condition for completion of graduate medical education. As we require the inclusion of identified subjects in the core psychiatric curriculum, we should require evaluation of our programs' capacity to impart that knowledge.

Existing Mechanisms

Within medicine, there are a variety of self-assessment and in-training opportunities. The majority of the other 20 specialties that offer society-sponsored, self-assessment examinations, allow residents to engage in such assessments. Specific, optional in-training exams are available during residency in over three-quarters of the specialties. (Several are available through specialty boards, specialty societies, or educational foundations or consortia.) Only two of the 24 major specialty areas—Allergy and Immunology, and Preventive Medicine—have neither self-assessments or in-training examinations.

The American Psychiatric Association offers a self-assessment program, Psychiatric Knowledge and Self-Assessment Program (PKSAP), available for APA members, other physicians, and residents; the American College of Psychiatrists offers an in-training examination, the Psychiatry Residency In-Training Examination (PRITE), available only to psychiatric residency programs. Neither of these programs, however, is designed or used to determine whether a resident has successfully completed training or to assess the quality of a particular residency program.

The only standardized indicator of skill and knowledge acquisition may be the American Board of Psychiatry and Neurology certifying examination. Because it can only be taken after completion of an approved residency program and satisfactory demonstration of credentials, it may serve as one means of assuring individual competency against a background of program diversity, but cannot be used for determining eligibility for graduation. Moreover, the ABPN exam is voluntary, and therefore may be taken several years after completion of residency. It tests skills acquired both during residency and in subsequent practice through continuing medical education, and is a seriously flawed substitute for in-service testing. As a solution, it has been suggested that the ABPN Part One written exam should be offered during the PGY-4 year, thereby serving the purposes of an in-service examination for both trainee and residency program. Countervailing arguments have been made that certification must remain separate from quality assurance program assessment, and that the purpose of ABPN certification would be compromised were the Part One exam offered during residency.

Developing an In-Service Examination

Given the complexities inherent in planning and implementing an in-service examination, it is appropriate to convene a consortium of concerned organizations (including but not limited to the APA, ABPN, American Association of Chairmen of Departments of Psychiatry, the American Association of Directors of Psychiatric Residency Training, the Association for Academic Psychiatry, and the American Academy of Child and Adolescent Psychiatry) to undertake this activity. Their product would be the establishment of a comprehensive examination upon which successful completion of the residency program would be predicated.

However, the development and implementation of a psychiatric in-service examination raises a host of questions which this consortium must address: When and how can we test for knowledge and skills needed in the care of physical illness and neurology? How are we to insure reliability, stability, and validity of the examination and, at the same time, provide feedback to both programs and those taking the examinations? How can we account for different sequences in training? Should we provide and can we afford to provide extended training for those found significantly deficient on in-service examinations?

Another obvious issue critical to the efficacy of this in-service examination is the nature of the instrument itself. Rather than a binary or multiple choice approach which tests only for cognitive knowledge, the examination must assess both skills and cognitive knowledge. One mechanism that accomplishes both assessment goals and accommodates variance in sequencing would be the annual use of the critical clinical incidents cognitive examination (CCICE) utilizing criterion-referenced scoring. Among the advantages of the CCICE are that it facilitates assessment of history taking, interviewing, decision-making, rapport and alliance building, mental status testing, differential diagnosis, problem solving, and triage strategies. The careful selection of critical clinical incidents would enable trainees to be assessed for performance with a variety of patients, age groups and modalities. Before graduation, a resident would have to pass the examination based upon consortium agreed-upon standards.

Conclusion

The development of an in-service examination will benefit both future psychiatric residents and residency programs. Strengths will be noted, and weaknesses corrected in both. However, as psychiatric educators, we should not rest our concerns solely upon the development and implementation of such an in-service examination process. We must evaluate our examinations continuously, expanding and upgrading our assessment strategies and mechanisms. At the same time, we must ensure that the in-service examination remains the first of a variety of mechanisms to ensure that professional skills are maintained and new knowledge is gained over a professional lifetime. Only in this way can we assure ourselves, the public, and the patients we serve that our trainees meet a standard that we all find acceptable.

22

THE CRITICAL INCIDENT METHOD: AN EVALUATION MODEL

Allan Tasman, M.D.

Ronald Rieder, M.D.

An important component of psychiatric education in the '90s will be the evaluation of psychiatric residents, including assessment of the skills, knowledge, and attitudes essential for psychiatric practice. These evaluations will be conducted through a series of formal examinations that include the assessment of clinical performance.

Examination techniques utilize a variety of formats, and include objective examinations, both written and oral; practical examinations, essay examinations, project assignments, observation reports, and attitudinal measures. Unfortunately, the most widely used evaluation techniques—multiple choice and essay examinations, patient management problems, and project assignments—provide a good measurement of knowledge, but have limited ability to predict clinical performance, since they are limited to assessment of a knowledge base, not attitudes or behaviors.

Oral examinations can simulate clinical performance, but they may not be reliable, as the artifacts of the testing situation may interfere with objective demonstration of clinical skills. Systematic and repeated non-invasive observation of performance can provide a more reliable assessment, since behaviors are evaluated over long intervals, and external influences are minimized. Nonetheless, concerns about reliability and consistency of direct observational assessment or resident performance may limit the utility of this technique as well.

Direct observation may be influenced by the presence of an evaluator which may affect the behavior of the trainee under observation as well as the behavior of the patient. Some of this limitation may be ameliorated through extensive contact with the resident (either over a longer period of time or in a multiplicity of settings) but may not be cost effective in terms of the significant amount of time which must be expended both by evaluator and evaluatee.

Another difficulty is the use of appropriate patient material. Oftentimes, clinical evaluations are subject to the availability of patients, and there may be a skew in the clinical syndromes presented, severity of illness, etc. Additionally, insufficient rater training or lack of clarity of expected behaviors and their ranking can lead to wide variation in reported outcome or inter-rater reliability. The Hawthorne effect also must be considered; the very presence of an evaluative interaction may change behavior.

The use of simulation as an evaluation technique may overcome some of the problems inherent in observation of performance or in a written examination. The simulation may be more objective, with a clearly defined patient intervention, with specific responses to the examinee intervention (for example, a patient with a certain diagnosis can be simulated with appropriate clinical signs and symptoms, laboratory findings, etc.) making the evaluation procedure less dependent on the vagaries of patient availability. Simulations tend to move from testing the knowledge base to considering attitudes, behaviors, skills, and problem solving ability. An example of a useful simulation for evaluation is the patient management problem. These may be difficult to construct and may be limited by the stated choices provided to the candidates from which they must choose.

The Critical Incident Method

One type of simulation, the critical incident technique, developed by Flanagan in the 1940s, utilizes performance-based evaluation of behaviors or incidents having special (critical) significance based on systematically defined criteria. The technique has been utilized as a reliable and valid way to determine clinical competence in a number of medical specialties and has found wide utility in industry and government. It is proposed here as an approach to performance appraisals of psychiatric residents. Flanagan defined these critical incidents as behaviors vital or central to care in a clinical situation; the technique refers to settings in which the consequences of the actions of the physician are easily observable. Thus, this type of simulation avoids the assessment of global skills sometimes used in evaluation checklists, such as reliability and conscientiousness. Rather, it focuses on very specific skills and behaviors demanded in a particular clinical situation.

The choice of the critical incident is vital to the success of the method. The incident must be sufficiently circumscribed to enable the observer to judge the impact of the behavior of the person engaged in the simulation, on the patient. At the same time, the consequences of the actions undertaken in the simulation must be definitive, leaving little doubt as to their effect.

The critical incident method was first used during World War II to understand why certain individuals failed in navy pilot training. The initial question asked was: "What makes a good or bad pilot?" Extensive interviews were conducted with trainers to determine the characteristics of people who succeeded and to obtain examples of their desired behaviors. The predictive value of the criteria developed from these interviews was then tested by evaluating people about to enter pilot training. The outcome or actual performance (of both those who completed training and those who were not successful) was then compared with performance on the evaluations.

Applying the critical incident method to psychiatric residents starts with a similar question. "What are the behaviors in what clinical situations that make a good psychiatrist?" While there are no agreed-upon specific national standards by which psychiatrists are judged, Langsley and Hollender's listing of the skills, knowledge, and attitudes essential to practice is a first step.

Considerable pre-planning is necessary to implement this technique. Essential steps include: determining the aim or objective of the specific evaluation, setting up the simulation including gathering and classifying data, and instructing the evaluators.

Developing a Critical Incident Evaluation Protocol

The first step in developing a protocol is to define the objective of the evaluation. Is it an evaluation for minimal overall clinical competence, or is it to identify outstanding behavior? What is the relationship of the outcome of the evaluation to resident promotion or graduation? A clear statement of its purpose and function, and, thus, the threshold for satisfactory outcome (passing) is vital.

Table 1. Observer's Comments

"Consulted with staff before saw patient"
"Kept appropriate physical distance"
"Had calm demeanor"
"Stood over patient while talking"
"Didn't hear the patient out"
"Seemed as upset as the patient"
"Suggested more medication right away"
"Gave patient time to tell his story"
"Threatened patient with seclusion"
"Did formal mental status exam"
"Helped patient reality test"
"Was firm but not angry"
"Didn't notice the patient was escalating"
"Too vague about what the patient should do"
"Asked for help when it seemed necessary"
"Let the patient know he understood his worries"
"Went to see patient initially with security guards"
"Asked too many unstructured questions"
"Let the patient know he wanted to help"
"Let the patient sign out right away"
"Found out what set off the patient"
"Jumped to conclusions too fast"
"Tried to put his hand on the patient"
"Spoke clearly and concretely to patient"
"Started by demanding the patient to calm down"
"Firmly told patient he needed help"
"Noticed when patient was escalating, and backed off"
"Too verbose, not concrete enough"

The next step is to set up the clinical simulation itself. Designated observers identify and agree upon a specific critical incident to be evaluated and determine what clinical situations are appropriate to examine discreet episodes with a scope of observable outcomes. Types of appropriate and inappropriate resident response within each identified clinical situation are enumerated. Observers then assess the relative importance of the particular resident behaviors in the context of an overall judgment of resident performance in each situation.

An example illustrating this method would be a critical incident in which a resident is called upon to assess a psychotic inpatient who is demanding to sign out against medical advice. The capacity to assess a patient's mental status is the skill of particular importance in this example. Observer comments based upon multiple observation of residents in this situation are outlined in Table 1.

The next step is to classify the data, based on the purpose of the evaluation. Table 2 shows how a first level of categorization might be obtained in the example cited above, if the question is to ascertain quality performance. For example, the resident's observational capacities should include the ability to gather data from staff and patient, to identify the patient's nonverbal behavior, and to notice patient changes occurring in the course of the interview. Ideally, these behaviors should be clearly and non-equivocally demonstrable such that the raters can agree as to their presence or absence.

Then there is further categorization or ranking to identify the most critical of behaviors. Table 3 illustrates how data can be classified according to the relative weight of specific positive and negative resident behaviors. For the purposes of this example, only one category, "Interventions," is considered. In actual use, each category would be subject to similar classification.

Yet another dimension of the evaluation is determining how critical a particular behavior is to the purpose of the evaluation itself. Table 4 provides an example of data critical to the goal of the evaluation for the "Interventions" category.

The overall classification of data will result in a checklist to be used in future resident evaluation. The necessary aspects of the checklist include: (1) that the heading structure be easily discernible; (2) that the categories be clinically meaningful; (3) that the items be stated neutrally; (4) that data groupings be weighted equally; and (5) that the headings be comprehensive.

The clarity and specificity of the identified behaviors will assist in examiner training and improve inter-rater reliability. Training of evaluators (who may or may not be the persons responsible for the initial data collection and ranking) is relatively straight forward. A simulated critical incident method development process was undertaken at a recent meeting of the American Association of Directors of Psychiatric Residency Training. Initial review of data from that simulation indicates surprisingly good consensus among participants, both in listing criteria to evaluate specific clinical situations, as well as in weighting aspects of resident performance.

Table 2. Classifying Data: "What Makes a Good Performance?"

I. OBSERVATIONAL

- Gathered data from staff and patient
- Identified patient's non-verbal behavior
- Noticed changes in patient while talking

II. ATTITUDINAL

- Empathic, let patient know he was aware of problem
- Calm, non-impulsive
- Firm in statement of treatment recommendations
- Communicated wish to be helpful

III. PHYSICAL BEHAVIOR

- Not intrusive—kept appropriate distance
- Not threatening—no unexpected changes in behavior

IV. VERBAL BEHAVIOR

- Clear and concise with patient
- Clear and concise with staff
- Provided reality testing
- Provided concrete structure for patient

V. INTERVENTIONS

- Focused on maintaining alliance
- Included staff in assessment
- Assessed need for continued hospitalization
- Assessed accurately need for medication
- Assessed need for seclusion-restraint
- Good communication of findings and plan to patient
- Good communication of findings and plan to staff

Table 3. Weighing the Data

A. Critical to Outcome of Incident

V. Interventions

Major
- focused on maintaining alliance
- assessed need for continued hospitalization
- assessed need for medication
- assessed need for seclusion/restraint

Minor
- included staff in assessment
- communicated findings and plan to patient
- communicated findings and plan to staff

Table 4. Classifying the Data

B. Critical to Purpose of Evaluation

If purpose is minimal competence at beginning of PGY-2

V. Interventions

Major
- focused on alliances
- assessed need for medication
- assessed need for hospitalization
- assessed need for seclusion

If purpose is average performance at end of PGY-2

V. Interventions

Major
- All categories

Summary

The critical incident method of evaluation has been shown to be well suited for evaluating clinical competence. The advantages of this form of assessment are: (1) as a simulation, it can examine behavior in specific, pre-set situations; (2) it evaluates behaviors across many aspects of performance; and (3) it evaluates complex behaviors involving a variety of motor and/or interpersonal components; (5) attitudes and interpersonal style, as well as skill mastery, can be assessed; and (5) it supports more reliable observations and conclusions.

The critical incident method can be used in the direct observation of resident-patient interaction. Since the technique relies on relatively simple judgments by qualified observers, based on a previously agreed-upon statement of purpose, supervisors and other educators can be more specific in formulating assessments of clinical performance. While substantial time is necessary to set up the method, once the data sheets are developed, the process is relatively simple, allowing educators to integrate the product of these assessments into the conduct of individual resident educational efforts and experiences in programs.

References

1. Langsley DG, Hollender M: The definition of a psychiatrist. Am J Psychiat 139:81-85, 1982
2. Strauss GD, Yager J, Strauss GE: Assessing assessment: The content and quality of the psychiatric in-training examination. Am J Psychiat 139:85-88, 1982
3. Strauss GD, Yager J, Liston EH et al: Testing psychiatric knowledge with in-house examinations. Am J Psychiat 138:636-641, 1981
4. Chevron ES, Rounsaville BJ: Evaluating the clinical skills of psychotherapists. Arch Gen Psychiat 40:1129-1137, 1983
5. Liston E, Yager J: Assessment of clinical skills in psychiatry, in Teaching Psychiatry and Behavioral Science. Edited by Yager J. New York, Grune and Stratton, 1982, pp. 515-528.
6. Segall AJ, et. al: Systematic Course Design for Health Fields, New York, J. Wiley and Sons, 1975
7. McGuire CH: The oral examination as a measure of professional competence. J Med Ed 41:267-274, 1966
8. Pokorny AD, Frazier SH: An evaluation of oral examinations. J Med Ed 41:28-40, 1966

9. Foster JT, Abrahamson S, Lass S, et al: Analysis of an oral examination use in specialty board certification. J Med Ed 44:951-954, 1969
10. Flanagan JC: The critical incident technique. Psychol Bull 51:327-358, 1954
11. Hubbard JP, Levit EJ, Schumacher CF et al: An objective evaluation of clinical competence. NEJM 272:1321-1328, 1965
12. Sanazaro PJ, Williamson JW: A classification of physician performance in internal medicine. J Med Ed 43:389-397, 1968
13. Levine HG, McGuire CH: Rating habitual performance in graduate medical education. J Med Ed 46:306-311, 1971
14. Newble DI, Hoare J, Elmslie RG: The validity and reliability of a new examination of the clinical competence of medical students. Med Ed 15:46-52, 1981
15. Newble DI: The critical incident technique: A new approach to the assessment of clinical performance. Med Ed 17:401-403, 1983
16. McDermott J, McGuire C, Berner E: Roles and functions of child psychiatrists, in Report on the Project on Certification of Child Psychiatry. Evanston, IL. American Board of Psychiatry and Neurology, 1976
17. Goleman D: The new competency tests: Matching the right people to the right jobs. Psychology Today, January 1986

PART 4:

RESIDENCY PROGRAM ACCREDITATION

Accreditation of psychiatric residency training is conducted by the Accreditation Council for Graduate Medical Education (ACGME) through the Residency Review Committee (RRC) for Psychiatry. The General Essentials of Accredited Residencies detail the requirements for all graduate medical education programs; the Special Requirements (Essentials) for Residency Training in Psychiatry, developed by the RRC for Psychiatry, describe the required form and content of psychiatry residency training programs.

In recent years, the RRC has codified more clearly the requirements for clinical training, specifying sites and rotation length for resident assignments. For example, to assure that training programs adequately prepare residents to work with severely ill patients, the RRC, through the Special Requirements, may require one year on inpatient services. Some programs argue that this plan hampers their capacity to train in sites, such as day hospitals, available within their clinical facilities. If all programs are obliged to provide a full year of inpatient rotation, a particular program might be unable to assign trainees to its day hospital, thereby excluding training in an important treatment locale. The RRC argues that without specific requirements, it cannot maintain appropriate minimal training standards.

Some educators see the process of site visits by which training programs are reviewed as the heart of the accreditation problem.

They argue that the RRC, using non-specialist site visitors, cannot properly inspect and review the programs it evaluates. These critics suggest that careful program examination by a psychiatrist/educator, rather than by a physician from another specialty, would enable the RRC to make better use of present rules and regulations. They argue further that the imposition of highly specific, detailed requirements limits the creativity that training directors may bring to the educational process, resulting in a downward leveling effect across all training programs.

A further question relates to the future role of subspecialization in psychiatric practice and training. If increasing subspecialization in practice mandates increased specialization in education, the imposition of specific Requirements (Essentials) will serve only to highlight programs that emphasize subspecialty training to the detriment of programs that do not.

What follows are two position papers. Cooper advocates RRC Special Requirements (Essentials) for Residency Training in Psychiatry that set goals and standards rather than the delineation of specific experiences and activities; Talbott suggests that it is the RRC's function to identify and regulate the minimal standards. He also argues that alternative training sites and innovative programming must be supported in order to meet future clinical needs while attending to economic realities.

Stefan Stein, M.D.

23

THE ROLE OF THE RESIDENCY REVIEW COMMITTEE: GENERAL PRINCIPLES FOR RESIDENCY PROGRAMS

Arnold M. Cooper, M.D.

The goals of the Residency Review Committee (RRC) for Psychiatry should be threefold: (a) to assure that psychiatry training programs maintain a minimal standard of psychiatric education; (b) to encourage these programs to achieve an optimal standard; and (c) to encourage the development of innovative psychiatry training programs and training faculty. Unfortunately, as the Special Requirements (Essentials) for Residency Training in Psychiatry are drawn today, emphasis is placed primarily upon meeting minimum standards of educational quality and content.

Because programs differ enormously in their clinical settings, patient populations, and available faculty resources, it is difficult for each to meet the same set of stringent standards. Thus, the RRC should develop a thoughtful document detailing core knowledge and skills around which individual programs may shape their own training programs. For example, rather than requiring a time-specified inpatient rotation, the RRC would be more wise to establish the range of skills, knowledge, and attitudes which are intended to be achieved during such an experience. Innovative program directors, then, could find ways to develop these required capabilities through the types of training experiences best provided in their individual institutions. Indeed, inpatient services are sufficiently varied, that their educational goals are already substantially heterogeneous.

There seems to be general agreement among psychiatric educators that we should be training for the future; yet there is little agreement upon precisely what the future holds for psychiatric practice. Under these circumstances, the wisest choice would be to rededicate our residencies toward broader educational concepts rather than more specific training. Training develops skills; the core skills required of the psychiatrist may be few, but they are difficult to master. Core skills, once acquired, are easily modified to meet new situations. For example, if a resident has mastered interviewing techniques, then relatively little additional training will be necessary to enable the psychiatrist to adapt to differing settings.

In preparing for an uncertain world, it is most important to emphasize the solid intellectual base of the profession and aid in the development of basic skills. Psychiatrists must learn both the history and the current state of knowledge in the major areas of the field: nosology, epidemiology, biology, psychodynamics, etc. Some aspects will be "old" knowledge; some will be rather new, representing developing, but now vital parts of psychiatry's armamentarium, such as pharmacology and genetics. Similarly, the uncertain future requires that young psychiatrists be able to continue learning and acquiring new knowledge, while being critical in the evaluation of these new areas. As education, in contrast to skills acquisition, assumes a more significant role in the residency, we should become more like university evaluators rather than trade school evaluators.

The current RRC Special Requirements (Essentials) meet few, if any, of the new realities of changing clinical settings, new research advances, changing technologies, and service needs. Rather than describing required exposure to every existing area of the field, the RRC should be attending more to faculty-student ratios, available mix of patient populations, and availability of library resources. The RRC components seem to reflect a need not to leave out one therapeutic modality, rather than to specify a hierarchical order of knowledge acquisition.

Current RRC Special Requirements (Essentials) encourage superficial learning in many areas, discouraging deep immersion, or excitement about the profession. Emphasis upon skills acquisition alone will only damage the educational process in the future. The RRC should develop a carefully limited set of required basic skills built upon a broad and deep knowledge base which set more realistic minimal standards for psychiatric education. By focusing on this core, the RRC will help programs ensure that graduates master enduring professional attitudes and competencies, even as the specific daily tasks of a psychiatrist take on new focus under new political and environmental requirements. The new requirements also will give greater impetus to the development of innovative residency programs and encourage the attainment of optimal, rather than minimal goals.

24

THE RESIDENCY REVIEW COMMITTEE: INCREASED DIVERSITY AND INNOVATION IN RESIDENCY TRAINING

John A. Talbott, M.D.

The founders of the American Psychiatric Association numbered only 13—now there are over 33,000 psychiatrists. The sole practice site for our forebearers was the freestanding mental hospital; today, psychiatrists practice in a variety of inpatient and outpatient settings. Originally, there was a single goal—clinical care; today psychiatrists may be equally skilled in clinical care, education, research, and health economics (1). Finally, while in the 19th century there were no "subspecialties" in psychiatry, today at least a dozen areas that can be considered specialties exist (2), although much variation exists with respect to "subspecialty" content and specificity.

History of the RRC

The increasing complexity of our field is reflected in the increased specificity included in the recent revision of the Residency Review Committee's Special Requirements (Essentials) for Residency Training in Psychiatry. The first of these guidelines was issued in 1952, and specified only the following:

> *The training for psychiatrists should include clinical work with psychoneurotic and psychotic patients, combined with the study of basic psychiatric sciences, medical and social psychology,*

> *psychopathology, psychotherapy and the physiological therapies, including a basic knowledge of the form, function and pertinent pathology of the nervous system. This training should be supervised and guided by teachers competent to develop skill and understanding in the utilization of such basic knowledge in dealing with patients. Mere factual knowledge is not sufficient. The training period should include instruction in the psychiatric aspects of general medical and surgical considerations and the behavior disorders of children and adolescents sufficient to develop practical ability to direct the treatment of such conditions. It should also include collaborative work with social workers, clinical psychologists, courts and other social agencies. The training program of the candidate for certification in psychiatry should include sufficient training in neurology to enable him to recognize and to evaluate the evidences of organic neurological disease* (3).

The most recent draft, 27 pages longer and worlds apart, requires knowledge in medicine as well as in 10 separate areas of psychiatry: major theories, biopsychosocial factors in development, psychiatric conditions, psychological assessment, financing and regulation, medical ethics, medical history, legal aspects, referrals, and research methods. Skills are specified in: clinical diagnosis, relation of findings to etiology and treatment, differential diagnosis, therapies, continuity of care, psychiatric consultation, administration, psychological testing, appraisal of the literature, and teaching. Residents' clinical experiences are expected to include a panoply of settings (inpatient, outpatient, community-based managed care, 24-hour emergency, and consultation-liaison service, substance abuse programs), and to crosscut patient age distinctions. Resident experiences must include exposure to neurological patients and to collaboration with other mental health personnel (4).

Thus, today's resident has a platter heaped high with requirements to complete during the post-graduate years. The training program is burdened by demands that may inhibit a more innovative, flexible approach, that could provide future residents with greater exposure to the emerging changes in population demographics, economics and services trends.

Future Trends

Major new findings in biomedical research will most certainly lead to dramatic changes in the practice of psychiatry. Our residency training programs are likely to accommodate readily to such new directions. Factors such as population trends, changing practice settings, and restructured health economics are more easily predicted, but much less likely to be reflected in training.

Demographic Trends

The next decade will mark the maturing of the post World War II baby-boom cohort into the age range when serious mental illness becomes manifest. The over-65 population will double by the year 2030. Both trends portend a steady shift in the ratio between the wage-earning and "dependent" populations; greater numbers will suffer from psychiatric illness and age-related mental impairments simply because there will be more people. The President's Commission on Mental Health in the late 1970s urged greater attention to the needs of underserved populations—the aged, children, minorities, and the chronically mentally ill, while the Graduate Medical Education National Advisory Committee (GMENAC) in 1980 reported an absolute shortage of psychiatrists (5). Efforts have been made to attract greater numbers of medical students into psychiatry, and to provide more comprehensive training to meet the needs of these underserved populations. Trends suggest, however, that our efforts must be redoubled.

Service Trends

The deinstitutionalization movement of the past two decades has moved the chronically mentally ill out of state hospitals in large numbers. While some patients have been integrated into outpatient treatment programs, others have become barely tolerated inmates of nursing homes or correctional facilities; still others have been found on the streets, numbered among the homeless. The role of psychiatric treatment in these newer settings is a service question of serious proportion.

Few residency programs have shifted the balance of their training as the balance of needed services has changed. We are simply not meeting the needs of psychiatric services in nursing homes, or jails, or in the cities' streets and shelters. A recent NIMH report asserted that there is not a single board-certified psychiatrist on staff full-time in any of the more than 2,000 skilled nursing facilities in this country (6). The RRC Special Requirements (Essentials) do not take into account the mechanisms that must be developed by our training programs to educate residents for these new settings.

Economic Trends

The economics of health care in the 1980s has been dominated by two camps that seem diametrically opposed: the cost containment movement and the corporate movement. At the very time that public policy makers have moved toward prospective pricing and the stimulation of competition through "new" entities such as HMOs, PPOs, IPAs and prudent buyer initiatives, the corporate sector has recognized psychiatry, and indeed all of medicine, as a profitable enterprise. Cost containment efforts place pressure on psychiatry not only by means of cost controls, but by increasing competition among physicians and from nonphysician practitioners. The corporatization of medicine places similar but opposite pressure upon our discipline to submerge individual practice to organized, vertically integrated corporate practice.

Few residency programs teach their trainees how to practice "as a group," and fewer still teach how to "market," to compete in a pro-competitive environment, or to survive in the world of corporate medicine. Health economists have posited that in the not-too-distant future the solo private practitioner will disappear, that most physicians will work for one of 8 to 10 corporate health giants, that as many as 10 percent of hospitals will close, and up to 10 percent of physicians will leave medical practice.

Last year, one-half of the graduating residents in one West Coast program went to work not in academic settings, as in the past, but in HMOs (7). Recent graduates have lamented the poor preparation given them in dealing with patients usually seen in community mental health centers—the retarded, the chronically mentally ill, and the substance abusers. These psychiatrists also express concern about the increased knowledge they need in administration, personnel, budget and finance.

These reports argue against maintaining the status quo in existing training programs and support the development of innovative curricula and training sites to prepare for an uncertain future.

The Argument For Innovative/Flexible Training

While we are better off teaching people how rather than what to think, we can teach our trainees to think as well in alternative settings as in our familiar hospitals. Indeed, there appears to be a direct relationship between residents' training experiences and their later choice of practice site and area of interest (8). If we foreclose training in other than traditional locations, we may well foreclose practice in other than these traditional settings.

While stressing how to think, we must equally promote how to practice, as well as where to practice, exposing trainees to multiple settings, practice patterns, and treatment modalities. By combining modern, formal curricular material in innovative practice settings, no type of setting or form of practice will seem unfamiliar.

The Dilemmas We Face

Even if we agree that the world is changing rapidly and irreversibly, that residents will not practice psychiatry how or where we do, and that training programs must offer more diversity of content and exposure, we have several unsolved problems.

First, funds still do not "follow" the patient from setting to setting. Inpatient reimbursement continues to "pay the freight" for most residency training programs, though this base of support may change as legislators tinker with direct and indirect cost payments for education under Medicare. From an administrator's perspective, inpatient care is more cost efficient to the program since other settings may not be subject to insurance reimbursement at all!

Second, "exposing" trainees to alternative settings, as suggested by the RRC Special Requirements (Essentials), is insufficient. We must offer training, supervision, and role models equal in quality to those found in "traditional" settings, reflecting differing styles of practice found in different types of milieu.

Conclusion

The RRC Special Requirements (Essentials) for Residency Training in Psychiatry might best be served by the addition of another prescriptive paragraph:

> *All of the above are the necessary elements of a good training program, elements which, in the final analysis, while necessary, are insufficient. The requirements must be put together with flexibility, innovation and excellence—in varied and innovative settings that offer the trainee exposure to a variety of practice styles and treatment programs. In addition, the goals of flexibility, innovation, and excellence take precedence over any specific item.*

The whole, then, must be greater than the sum of the parts, and the outcome, an increased ability to prepare trainees for a rapidly changing future.

References

1. Talbott JA: Contemporary social issues and decisions that will affect the future practice of psychiatry, in De Rerum Futura: The Measure of Psychiatry in the '80s and Beyond. Edited by Freidel R. Pfizer/Roerig, in press
2. Talbott JA, Granet RB: Careers in psychiatry: Options for the future. Comprehen Psychiat 25:263-277, 1984
3. Medical Specialties: American Board of Psychiatry and Neurology: Specialized training. JAMA 150:411-412, 1952
4. Special requirements for residency training in psychiatry. Accreditation Council for Graduate Medical Education. August 29, 1985 (draft)
5. Office of Graduate Medical Education, Health Resources Administration: Report of the Graduate Medical Education National Advisory Committee. Washington, DC, DHHS Pub. HRA-81-652, 1980
6. Harper M, Lebowitz B (Eds.): Mental Illness in Nursing Homes: Agenda for Research. Rockville MD, National Institute of Mental Health, 1986
7. Lanman R, personal communication
8. Langsley DG, Robinowitz CB: Psychiatric manpower: An overview. J Hosp Comm Psychiat 30:749-755, 1979
9. Talbott JA, Sharfstein SS: A proposal for future funding of chronic and episodic mental illness. J Hosp Comm Psychiat, in press
10. Granet RB, Perry SW, Talbott JA: A resident's rotation in consultation psychiatry: A maturational experience. Gen Hosp Psychiat 2:306-309, 1980
11. Weintraub W, Harbin HT, Book J, et al: The Maryland plan for recruiting psychiatrists into public service. Am J Psychiat 141:91-94, 1984

PART 5:

FINANCING RESIDENCY TRAINING

Of fundamental concern for the future of psychiatric education have been the economic factors that will change the sources and structure of funding. These will require adaptation and creativity on the part of those responsible for training. There is no longer an expectation for stable funding sources. Training directors and department chairmen often must make arrangements that they feel will threaten the integrity and direction of their programs.

Goldman, Sharfstein and Stein, in their chapter, detail the changes that have occurred and describe those on the horizon. They recommend several options, emphasizing the need for collaboration between the private and public sectors, and suggesting the development of an all-payer mechanism to spread the cost of medical education equitably. Webb and Beigel, noting that economic realities must be reflected in the "content and conduct" of residency training programs, believe that "financing changes should not determine the focus of future psychiatric education." They advocate for continuing attention to training residents to care for chronic and long-term patients and for sensitivity to the ethical and pragmatic problems they will face in the future.

In his chapter on the impact of economic factors on undergraduate medical education, Kay focuses on the dilemmas facing faculty who are required to generate their salaries through clinical reve-

nues, and may be less available to teach. He suggests that residents will play an important role in future undergraduate medical education in psychiatry.

Carol C. Nadelson, M.D.
Carolyn B. Robinowitz, M.D.

25

NEW REIMBURSMENT MODELS AND RESIDENCY TRAINING: THE CHANGING CLINICAL AND EDUCATIONAL FUTURE

Steven S. Sharfstein, M.D.

Howard H. Goldman, M.D.

Stefan Stein, M.D.

The end of World War II ushered in the modern era of medical education and specialty training. Growing recognition of the prevalence of mental disorders nationwide and the inadequate numbers of psychiatrists to meet population needs culminated in passage of the National Mental Health Act in 1946. This Act, establishing the National Institute of Mental Health (NIMH), mandated expansion of the supply of psychiatrists by providing direct training support to hospitals and medical schools.

Since 1946, largely through the impetus of the NIMH, the number of psychiatrists has increased nearly tenfold; patient care episodes in the specialty mental health system have quadrupled. Further, psychiatric care settings have become substantially more diversified, now including psychiatric units in general hospitals, community mental health centers, and office practice in private settings (1).

The 1980s have brought additional changes in the wake of changing health care policy. Manpower needs are no longer a central focus. We have moved from an era in which some flexible, but "soft" federal money was available from the NIMH to support psychiatric manpower education, to an era in which little, if any, support from the NIMH can be anticipated. Today, cost containment is the highest priority not only for the federal government, but also for state and local governments. This priority affects public and private sector medical care in general, and psychiatry in particular.

Third-party insurance historically has discriminated against patients with psychiatric disorders by not reimbursing their care in the same way as other medical care. There has been even greater constriction in public and private insurance programs in recent years. These trends, coupled with more recent federal efforts to control health care costs, have limited subsidies for graduate medical education. Market-based, competitive strategies to contain health care costs require academic health care facilities and other training sites to adhere to new rules and expectations (2). These competitive strategies also require medical educators, including psychiatrists, to consider changes in residency curricula to ensure that future practitioners are well versed in health economics and prepared to practice in new ways and under new structures.

Medicare and Financing Graduate Medical Education

In the past, the costs of residency training programs were underwritten by a variety of mechanisms. As noted by Nadelson and Robinowitz, training was financed predominantly through cross-subsidization by service fees. The expenses associated with running a teaching service were regarded as part of the "cost of doing business" and included in cost based financing mechanisms. Hospitals generally funded training by a pass-through factored into the hospital's charges for patient care. This factor included both direct costs of resident stipends, fringe benefits, and faculty salaries; and indirect costs (including increased use of laboratory tests and longer patient stays brought about by the training mission of the institution). These costs were then passed on to health care payers. This practice was accepted by all parties involved in financing medical treatment and by public policy makers, and justified on the grounds that high quality medical training was a necessary social good. Nowhere was this more evident than in the federal Medicare payment system.

As the cost containment agenda for health care became a dominant theme in the late 1970s and early 1980s, the efficacy of such cross-subsidization was called into question in public policy debate. Was this the most efficient way to finance medical education? Does cross-subsidization inappropriately mask the true cost of training? Should everyone continue to subsidize training, or should trainees or training institutions, the direct financial beneficiaries of the specialized training pay an increased share?

Driven by a desire to hold down Medicare expenditures, Congress enacted a change in direct and indirect hospital payments for graduate medical education as part of the Prospective Payment System (PPS) for Medicare under the Social Security Amendments of 1983. Graduate medical education is no longer subsidized by being billed as part of overall treatment charges. Payment for treatment has been capped through the introduction of Diagnosis Related Groupings (DRGs) into which patient admissions are categorized and under which reimbursement is calculated, not by actual expense or service but by predetermined formulae. The direct cost of graduate medical education may be passed through, but it is calculated far more tightly, based upon the number of full time equivalent (FTE) residents in training multiplied by the proportion of Medicare patients in the facility. Indirect costs have been capped at a fixed percentage. The era of educational financing through cross-subsidization under Medicare has ended.

Since adoption of the PPS, however, cries of injustice have been heard. Some public sector, urban academic-center institutions are being hard hit by PPS in direct proportion to their caseload of severely ill, labor-intensive and indigent care patients. These institutions find graduate medical education payments to be important in covering costs. Critics also have argued that many hospitals that are considered "teaching hospitals" are being subsidized excessively and inappropriately by other hospitals. The "teaching hospital" category also includes many community hospitals that do a small amount of teaching. Their overall costs are not substantially above the average since their case mix is not skewed toward the high-cost patient. In a sense, then, although some teaching facilities are losing money, others are receiving "double benefits," in both direct and indirect subsidy of their teaching programs. Their patient care costs are actually covering the expenses of their medical education programs, yet they receive the supplementary direct pass-through and the indirect fixed-dollar payments simply because they are "teaching hospitals." The considerable differential between the cost of providing routine care in a community hospital and a university hospital is not fully reflected in the PPS. Many remedies have been proposed. These include eliminating the indirect payment, changing the definition of "teaching hospital," changing the indirect payment formula, and placing a limit on the direct medical education pass-through. These and other mechanisms are currently under consideration by the U.S. Congress and the Administration. The ultimate adoption of federal solutions to the dilemma of Medicare financing for graduate medical education through service financing mechanisms will have important implications for the financing of medical education under other federal programs such as the Public Health Service Act (3) and upon private sector educational initiatives.

Paying for Training: Private Sector Options

In a time of cost conscious providers and price conscious payers and consumers, everything that is not directly profitable is being cut. Budget horizons do not extend beyond a year or two at the most; neither research nor training reaps an immediate profit. The content of training programs is antithetical to the emphases of prospective pricing and mechanisms that provide sharp incentives for efficiency, reduced length of stay, and limited intervention and laboratory testing. Equally, the increased resource needs typical of the severely ill, who are the referral caseload of teaching hospitals, are not easily accommodated by the prospective pricing systems being adopted by private third-party payers and by closed-panel, prepaid health plans.

The majority of hospitals operating under these new economic conditions are not teaching institutions and, as a result, they have lower costs to be passed through to third-party insurers or patients. These facilities have an advantage in setting rates and negotiating contracts, since they avoid the added burdens of teaching costs. Similarly, Health Maintenance Organizations (HMOs), able to reduce costs by eliminating training from their programs, also are able to deliver care more cheaply, placing university teaching facilities at an economic disadvantage in the private-payer market. A crucial question will be whether third-party payers consider it in their self-interest to subsidize the increased cost of training new physicians and specialists. If not, we could see a collapse in the "market" for teaching programs.

The rise of for-profit, investor-owned hospital chains provides an interesting opportunity for teaching hospitals in this cost competitive era. A number of these institutions have begun to lease or purchase university teaching hospitals as "flagships," vertically integrating their systems by first training physicians and then providing jobs for their graduates. The acquisition of teaching facilities also helps the investor-owned corporations improve their public image and obtain greater access to tertiary care. The extent to which these arrangements will continue, and the degree to which they provide a full range of clinical training experiences are issues not yet resolved.

A variety of public policy options that explicitly take into account the added costs of training should be explored. These include a specific "medical education" tax on third-party payers or on providers, and/or the development of program guidelines to pay for training costs for specific numbers of years, or specific specialties or subspecialties.

Options for Funding Graduate Medical Education

With major changes taking place in how we pay for medical care, we also must think through the closely related questions of how we pay for psychiatric residency training, where that training will occur, and whether the product will meet both public need and professional caliber. Economic realities dictate new approaches to graduate medical education. Two significant departures from current thinking offer more wide-ranging mechanisms to balance cost against public good. Whether the profession can ensure that the quality of education can be maintained under these or other new systems which may be adopted will be a challenge.

The establishment of a universal public insurance mechanism would avoid cross-subsidization of all kinds throughout the health care delivery system. All forms of hospital cost shifting, whether from private paying patient to public patient (skimming), from teaching cost to treatment cost, from hospital cost to nursing home cost (dumping), become more difficult in an all-payers system where everyone plays by the same set of financing rules. Special needs for chronic care, for high technology, high cost treatment, and treatment by specialists can be accommodated in such a system. An all-payers mechanism for financing services also could develop a direct subsidy for medical education, conceptualizing it as a "user's tax" for research and development. It becomes an investment in the future of medical care.

The most comprehensive option for public financing of post-secondary education, but one laden with serious public policy questions beyond the scope of this paper, would be financial support in exchange for universal public service. Such a system would include either military or civilian placement for a fixed period of service. For physicians, this service would be deferred until the completion of medical training. Such a system could balance the societal cost with the societal benefit of a public investment in medical post-graduate education. The proposal raises other questions about funding of this service.

Conclusion

Medical educators must help policy makers strike a balance between today's profits and future benefits, direct and indirect payments, and inefficient service delivery and the cost of graduate medical education. We have an obligation to bring to light the broader social good of public health issues such as care of the indigent and the chronically mentally ill, and not to focus exclusively on economic issues which fail to address these issues. Equally, our training programs must balance the comprehension of economic realities and concerns about our patients' social welfare and the quality of care we deliver.

References

1. Foley HA, Sharfstein SS: Madness and Government: Who Cares for the Mentally Ill. Washington DC, American Psychiatric Press, Inc, 1983
2. Sharfstein SS, Beigel A: Less is more? Today's economics and its challenge to psychiatry. Am J Psychiat 141:1403-1408, 1984
3. Final Report of the AAMC Committee on Financing Graduate Medical Education: Financing Graduate Medical Education. Washington DC, Association of American Medical Colleges, 1986

26

THE NEW ECONOMICS AND THE CONTENT OF PSYCHIATRIC TRAINING

William Webb, M.D.

Alan Beigel, M.D.

Psychiatry, perhaps unknowingly, has already begun to reshape the conduct of practice to reflect the economic exigencies of the times. It has responded to the complex public policy interplay among professionals, consumers, and payers which has redirected the future of health care delivery. Because psychiatric residency training continues to provide the skills and experience necessary for future practice, psychiatric educators must integrate these economic realities into the content and conduct of residency training programs. However, these financing changes should not determine the focus of future psychiatric education, nor should they become the focus.

New systems of care delivery place a premium on the "bottom line," viewing the physician as a technician. As traditional reimbursement arrangements have changed, some training programs have been too quick to look for and accept clinical placements in settings inappropriate to the training mission, leading to unfulfilled promises of clinical care and incomplete training curricula. We must continue to view our task as that of educating professionals; we cannot restrict artifically either our training or our clinical affiliations based solely upon market economics. Whatever technical expertise we teach must be accompanied by appropriate theoretical understanding, provided in an atmosphere that promotes professional growth.

To that end, we should not abandon the Special Requirements (Essentials) for Residency Training in Psychiatry of the Residency Review Committee for Psychiatry (RRC) which stress that training must preserve didactic and clinical experiences. We should continue to emphasize an open and inquiring attitude toward new developments in diagnosis and treatment. Tomorrow's psychiatrists should have a full appreciation of the biological, psychological, and social aspects of mental disorders and other medical illnesses, as well as a humane and empathic understanding of patients.

The profession holds to the RRC Special Requirements (Essentials) that psychiatrists know how to perform psychotherapy, and that they have exposure to a range of psychotherapies. As noted elsewhere in this volume, psychiatrists are no longer the sole providers of this treatment modality. In fact, today's new economically driven health plans, predominantly Health Maintenance Organizations (HMOs) and other capitated programs, favor the nonpsychiatrist mental health professional as a less costly alternative to the psychiatrist for these treatments. Nonetheless, we should not abandon training in psychotherapy to keep current with the cost/reward system. Learning psychotherapy also contributes significantly to the emotional maturation of trainees and sensitizes the training psychiatrist to the care and empathic understanding of others—a central feature of professional identity. At the same time, however, it is our responsibility to make residents aware of the financial realities surrounding the practice of psychotherapy, of the competition from nonphysician mental health practitioners, and from other nonpsychiatrist physicians.

Another theme of the Special Requirements (Essentials) for Residency Training in Psychiatry is the trainees' exposure to and responsibility for a broad spectrum of patients in different age groups, diagnostic categories, and social circumstances. Many of the new delivery systems stress short-term, time-limited interventions; they do not emphasize care of the most severely ill. The focus on brief therapy does not imply that we should do away with long-term, continuous therapeutic experience for our residents. This type of care provides learning experiences unavailable in short-term intervention, giving a picture of the natural history of disease, adaptation and coping of patients, patient management, and other aspects of care.

Our training programs should not abandon experiences with the long-term patient because of reimbursement strategies. Rather, psychiatric educators and leaders should work with policy makers to redefine public policy to meet the treatment needs of the chronically mentally ill. Both public and private financial resources can support the clinical needs of this population; we must continue to train our residents to meet those needs. We should provide residents with knowledge of reimbursement options and roadblocks, encouraging innovative means of treating long-term patients within the new economic order.

Conclusion

Our trainees cannot be educated in a vacuum that dismisses changes in health economics. Greater emphasis must be placed on management, cost analysis, and new systems of delivery, not as a focus of clinical care per se, but as an additional area of skills acquisition necessary to practice psychiatry in the next decade. Care must be taken to sensitize trainees to a host of ethical issues arising from the new economics of health care—issues of double agentry, scarce resources, and medico-legal jeopardy.

The real question is not how programs can refocus their teaching based on economic pressures, but rather how the essential elements of training can be accomplished in a time of diminishing resources, how economic realities can be integrated into high quality service and education. Only by a continued focus on quality of the training experience, not just the vicissitudes of the economic marketplace, can we maintain our professional integrity.

27

NEW ECONOMIC ISSUES AND THE UNDERGRADUATE CURRICULUM

Jerald Kay, M.D.

In an evocative commentary, Guggenheim and Nadelson addressed the future uncertainty of our academic discipline (1). They elucidated the impact of diminishing federal and local support to departmental budgets on the morale and professional and educational activities of both psychiatric faculty and residents. They also spoke of the impact of these changes upon the quality of medical student education programs. With increasing demands for salary generation, reimbursement, and profits, faculty will likely be less available for traditionally valued teaching and scholarly activities. This viewpoint was recently supported by Stein, who told members of the National Health Lawyers Association, "So many changes lie ahead for faculty practice plans, that someday, working at a medical school will be a lot like working at IBM." He remarked further that the "job [of the practice planning manager] is to harness physicians so that they will be more efficient in a era of shrinking resources" (2).

Recently, many financially related concerns about the quality of medical student programs were also expressed by the directors of medical student education in psychiatry. In a late 1984 questionnaire to the Association of Directors of Medical Student Education in Psychiatry (ADMSEP), the Committee on Medical Student Education of the APA requested ADMSEP member views of the major problems in psychiatric medical student education. Seven of the ten highest ranked problems identified by the respondents were intimately connected with the overcommitment of psychiatric faculty and the decrease or loss of support for educational programs. Specifically, the directors identified some their most pressing problems as: not enough teachers; overworked, burned out, and poorly motivated faculty; lack of support, recognition, tenure, and monetary reward for committed teachers; and insufficient funding for psychiatric undergraduate medical education (3).

The survey results prompted this author, through the APA Committee on Medical Student Education, to investigate further the impact of changing realities and economics on undergraduate psychiatric programs. This second survey sought to uncover information regarding increasing faculty practice plan obligations and changing psychiatric resident participation in medical student teaching programs.

Methodology

This second survey, a 22-item questionnaire, was mailed by the APA Committee on Medical Student Education to the 117 members of the Association of Directors of Medical Student Education in Psychiatry (ADMSEP) in February 1985. The survey requested demographic questions (academic title, medical school, faculty status, number of hours per week spent on their job, tenure status, age, sex, length of service as director of medical education, among others). In addition, data were collected on faculty participation in practice plans or other mechanisms to tap private practice income. Respondents were asked to indicate how long the plan had been in effect, its ownership, disbursement mechanisms, and plan characteristics. Other questions inquired about practice plan benefits, changes in practice plan obligations over time, and whether plan obligations had an effect on time for research and scholarly pursuits, and on the medical student program.

The last two questions on the survey inquired about the effect of decreased NIMH training funds on their medical student education program, and the change, if any, in the amount of resident participation in these programs.

Results and Recommendations

Eighty-six (74 percent) of the 117 directors of medical student education in psychiatry completed the questionnaire. Approximately one-third of the respondents were each at the assistant, associate or full professor ranks (Table 1).

Table 1. Characteristics of Questionnaire Respondents (N = 86)

Characteristic		Percentage	
Academic Title			
Professor		30.2	
Associate Professor		30.2	
Assistant Professor		27.9	
Other		11.9	
Practice Site			
State University		56.5	
Private University		42.4	
Academic Status	All	State	Private
Full-time	64.3	74.5	54.3
Geographic full-time	27.4	19.1	34.3
Part-time	6.0	2.1	11.4
Volunteer	1.2	2.1	0
Other	1.2	2.1	0

Nearly 57 percent of the directors were employed by state universities. The mean number of hours worked per week was 44. The mean age of the prediminantly male directors was 45, and they had held their position for a mean of just over 7 years. The directors' time was spent about equally in direct medical student and resident teaching, and research, with considerably more time devoted to administrative and patient care activities (Table 2). Seventy directors (81 percent) reported participation in a university-based practice plan. (This group differed from other respondents across a number of variables: they were more senior (tenured), spent a greater number of hours per week on the job, and were more often employed by a state university.)

Most of these practice plans had been established for almost 10 years; 40 percent of the respondents indicated that the medical school owned the plan. Nearly one-fourth of the plans were departmentally owned.

The extent to which faculty participated in a practice plan in large measure was determined by the financial incentives to engage in such a plan. These incentives range widely, from plans which segregate professorial salary from practice plan earnings to

Table 2. Distribution of Time by Respondents

Mean Hours per Week Spent in Activity	All	State	Private
Medical Student Education	6.13	6.48	5.78
Psychiatric Resident Supervision	5.61	5.79	5.64
Administration	12.27	11.17	13.81
Patient Care	16.46	15.81	16.72
Research	5.03	5.02	5.14
Scholarly Activities	3.61	3.17	4.45

plans which link salary directly to practice plan earnings. Ten percent of the sample belonged to practice plans that had no financial incentive for practice (income is independent of level of earnings); those from private medical schools were more than twice as likely to be in such a plan. Seventeen percent of the sample, all but one of whom were employed by state universities, responded that their plan had no strong incentive to practice (income is relatively independent of level of earnings, except for annual adjustment). The largest percentage of the sample indicated their practice plan had an incentive to practice (although no minimum amount of practice income is required, and they are allowed to keep a portion of the income earned). Again, there was considerable difference between those in private institutions compared to state universities. Finally, nearly 16 percent of the sample belonged to a practice plan with a strong incentive to practice (in order to earn a specified portion of their salary, they were required to treat patients) (Table 3).

Sixty-five percent of survey participants indicated that between 1982 and 1985, there had been an approximate 10 percent increase in the number of patients they were required to see to fulfill their practice plan obligations. Not surprisingly, nearly 50 percent of these directors responded that the more rigorous practice obligations had an impact on the quality of students' programs; 75 percent of those responding believed there was less time available for teaching students. Eighty-eight percent of the directors also indicated that they had less time for scholarly and research activities; half reported increasing difficulty with professional advancement. The survey highlighted other changes affecting psychiatric education: twenty-five percent of the directors felt that trainees were working with fewer lower socioeconomic patients and that the patient population, in general, represented a more narrow range of diagnostic categories. Nearly 60 percent of directors suggested that NIMH funding curtailments have had an adverse effect, especially

Table 3. Practice Plan Characteristics

	Percentages		
Characteristic	All ($N = 70$)	State ($N = 43$)	Private ($N = 25$)
No incentive to practice	10.0	7.0	16.0
No strong incentive	17.1	25.6	4.0
Incentive—income independent	27.1	20.9	40.0
Incentive—must see patients	12.9	14.0	12.0
Strong incentive (keep $)	10.0	11.6	8.0
Strong incentive (to ceiling)	15.7	14.0	12.0
Flat contributions required	2.9	4.7	0.0
Other	4.3	2.3	8.0

Table 4. Effect of Decreased NIMH Funding

Response	No. of Programs ($N = 80$)	Percentage
Great positive effect	12	15
Moderate positive effect	4	5
Little positive effect	1	1
No effect	14	18
Little negative effect	11	14
Moderate negative effect	29	36
Great negative effect	9	8

Table 5. Prevalence of Increased Resident Participation in Medical Student Education

Response	All ($N = 68$)	State	Private
Yes	50% (34)	51.2% (21)	48% (12)
No	50% (34)	48.8% (20)	52% (13)

related to the loss of (1) summer fellowships (traditionally an important vehicle for identifying and nurturing those students interested in the field); (2) production and purchase of audio-visual aids; (3) innovative pilot projects; and (4) ability to reward excellent teachers (Table 4).

One half of the respondents reported an increase in resident participation in medical student teaching programs (Table 5). They attributed this change more to greater appreciation for the resident as teacher and increased resident interest in teaching, rather than to decreased educational funding or increased faculty practice plan obligations (Table 6).

The most important finding is that directors of medical student education estimated that over the last three years, there has been a small increase (approximately 8 percent) in the amount of time spent and the number of patients they have been required to treat to fulfill practice plan obligations. Neither this increase nor the modest 11 percent increase in income generated were as great as anticipated in the literature (1, 4). However, practice plan obligations were seen to have an effect on the availability of faculty to teach and the total amount of time available for students.

The articulated concern about the availability of time for research and scholarly activities raises questions about whether faculty are actually spending their professional time as they had planned. While issues of faculty morale and professional development were beyond the scope of this survey, one survey respondent's comment is salient:

There is a great deal of pressure now on faculty to produce income from practice. We adapt by using more part-time unpaid faculty, more residents, and we work harder. The effect on the motivation for teaching, and on the climate needed for scholarly and thoughtful teaching, however, is very noticeable. There are no more professors of psychiatry who have excellence in teaching as their major commitment. Instead, we grab an hour here and there.

As was noted in the earlier Committee on Medical Student Education study, the loss of NIMH undergraduate training support has had a much more significant effect on many programs than have practice plan obligations. Forty-four respondents provided additional comments about the specific effects of this funding change on their programs affecting both trainee programming and faculty finances.

On a more optimistic note, however, residents appear to be more active in student teaching both because of greater faculty appreciation for the capacity of the resident-teacher and increased resident interest in teaching. The valuable, even central contributions of residents to clinical clerkship experiences have been well documented (5). Residency training programs might offer organized instruction in teaching for residents, including large and small group experiences, as well as individual supervision.

Conclusion

Faculty practice plans began developing in the late 1960s at a time when medical school budgets increased dramatically (from $319 million in 1959 to $7.2 billion in 1983). These plans were required to support a new system with many more full-time faculty than in previous years. Physician-researchers and teachers were able to secure reasonably balanced academic positions by performing modest amounts of clinical work.

While only future surveys will discover whether these findings persist over time, the results of this survey support the need for

Table 6. Reasons for Increased Resident Participation in Medical Student Education

Reason	All ($N = 34$)	State	Private
Decreased Funding	3	2	1
Increased Practice Plans	9	5	4
Greater Appreciation for Resident-Teacher	28	18	10
Better Quality of Resident-Teacher	14	9	5
Increased Resident Interest in Teaching	21	12	8

vigilance, lest the impact of practice plans on faculty teaching time lead to a deterioration in the quality of medical student programs. This would have important implications for recruitment and retention of both residents and faculty. The student's experiences in the clinical curriculum may be altered by the changing patient population and the shift toward ambulatory care at the expense of inpatient care.

With dwindling financial support for medical education, however, there may be an evolving compromise to our previously established academic teaching environment. The solutions to these emerging economic problems require national, regional, institutional and departmental efforts.

References

1. Guggenheim FG, Nadelson CN: Earn-as-you-go pressures in academic psychiatry. Am J Psychiat 141:1571-1573, 1984
2. Cavanaugh SA, Kay J: Problems in undergraduate medical education in psychiatry. J Psychiat Ed (in press)
3. Reilley P: Significant Changes Seen for Faculty Practice Plans to Boost Income for Schools. AMA News, May 11, 1984
4. Chin D, et al: The relation of faculty academic activity to financing sources in a department of medicine. NEJM 312:1029-1034, 1985
5. Orleans CS, Houpt JL, Larson DB: Interpersonal factors in the psychiatry clerkship: New findings. Am J Psychiat 137:1101-1103, 1980

28

SUMMARY AND CONCLUSIONS: FUTURE DIRECTIONS

Carol C. Nadelson, M.D.

Carolyn B. Robinowitz, M.D.

The authors of this volume have reaffirmed the need to strengthen the quality of residency training at all levels, from the application process through outcome evaluation. They have emphasized the integration of the increased scientific knowledge base and technological advances into graduate education, and have advised reformulating the core curriculum to take these changes into account.

They have stressed that the resident should gain basic skills and understanding that can be transferred as new settings and approaches emerge.

The authors noted the impact of economic forces on educational programs as well as on health care delivery, and urged continued vigilance regarding quality of care and education within the constraints of new funding demands.

They also agreed that residency training programs should be directed by a psychiatrist responsible for all aspects of planning, implementation, monitoring, and evaluation of the major activities of trainees.

Selection and Admission

The authors agreed that:

- Psychiatric residency training programs should select the highest quality applicants by a process that is agreed upon by all participants and known to all applicants.

Training Settings

The primary goal of residency training is to produce competent professionals who can function in a variety of clinical settings. It is the responsibility of the training director and faculty to judge proposed training sites primarily, but not exclusively, on the basis of how they facilitate attaining the goals of the training process.

- Proposed settings need to be evaluated on multiple criteria, including whether they provide opportunities for the resident to acquire an adequate data base in a nurturant environment, with adequate role models/supervisors available; and whether there is congruence between the task and the supervisors.

In addition to traditional sites of training, there is a need for training in newer practice settings such as Health Maintenance Organizations (HMOs), as well as in non-traditional health care settings and those affected by different economic and societal constraints, such as community mental health centers, correctional systems, the Veterans Administration, military, Indian health services, and others. Exposure to every type of setting in every program was not considered essential.

In each of these settings, faculty must be involved actively in the planning, supervision, and evaluation of residents.

- There should be agreed upon faculty-to-resident ratios in each setting, as well as evidence of adequate accessibility of the faculty to residents.

In order to assure the highest quality of faculty commitment to the ongoing process of education throughout professional careers,

- there should be documented evidence of professional growth of the faculty as represented by scholarship, research, professional attainment, and public service.

Core Knowledge and Skills

The psychiatrist of the 1990s should be able to function in different settings and with different patient populations. It is essential to define core knowledge and skills, and to ensure that this base is acquired during the course of the residency, although not necessarily at one site. The authors:

- Affirmed the essential role of psychotherapy in the training of psychiatrists, with both shortand long-term experience, in a biopsychosocial approach to treatment.

They recommended that:

- Residents should be fully capable of assessing and making appropriate referrals of psychiatric patients in at least the following categories: children, adolescents, elderly, chronically ill, alcoholic patients and substance abusers, and medically and surgically ill patients who have psychiatric problems.
- More emphasis should be placed upon psychiatric residents working collaboratively with primary care physicians and mental health professionals.
- Increased research opportunities should be developed for residents. All psychiatric residents should have a required experience in planning and/or conducting empirical research, and research-intensive departments of psychiatry should have a formal track for residents interested in research careers. These departments should serve as regional resources, collaborating with other departments in their geographic area to enable interested and qualified residents to pursue these tracks.
- Program curricula also should include training in the use of computers, video and telecommunications and provide residents with an understanding of issues surrounding the economic aspects of health care.

Resident and Program Evaluation

To ensure that residency training programs produce high quality practitioners, the authors made a number of recommendations:

- Evaluation of psychiatric residency programs should be done only by a team of psychiatrists expert in psychiatric education.
- In addition to annual, formal, ongoing clinical evaluation, a written cognitive examination regarding critical clinical inci-

dents should be developed; passage of this examination should be necessary before graduation from a residency program.

- In-service training examinations, including the Psychiatric Residency In-Training Examination (PRITE), should be reserved for individual and program assessment, and for remediation.
- Residents should maintain a log of clinical experiences in sufficient detail to assure that minimum requirements are being met. Patient examples from the log should be used as part of the annual evaluation of clinical skills. The log must be reviewed by faculty.

Unresolved Issues

Major areas of debate that did not come to closure were the issues of subspecialization and supply of psychiatrists. Although the explosion of the knowledge base in psychiatry makes it impossible for residents to obtain expertise in all areas, there is no clear agreement as to how residents should gain needed subspecialty experience during the training period. While there is danger of fragmentation, the authors agreed that subspecialty training should be integrated into the final year of residency, and agreed that all residents may receive in-depth training in a particular area such as consultation-liaison or substance abuse. Some psychiatrists will choose to practice as generalists, others will shape their practice around a subspecialty interest and expertise.

Conclusion

While suggesting a variety of directions for the future of academic psychiatry and the shape of residency programs in the 1990s, the volume highlights the need for psychiatric educators to remain flexible in the face of uncertain directions in public policy making for medical care in general, and psychiatric education, in particular. The challenge to the profession to produce young psychiatrists who can both remain current with major scientific advances and meet the economic, service and quality assurance demands of forces outside psychiatry is formidable. Implementation of the foregoing recommendations may help psychiatry meet that challenge.

APPENDIX 1

THE RALEIGH CONFERENCE: WORK GROUP RECOMMENDATIONS AND DISCUSSION

PROGRAM PLANNING: TRAINING MODELS

Presenters: Donald G. Langsley, M.D.
Zebulon Taintor, M.D.

Facilitator: Jeffrey Houpt, M.D.

Reporter: James Hilliard, M.D.

Conference participants were in agreement that the current approach to psychiatric training, comprised of clinical experiences, supervision, and didactic seminars, will remain at the core of resident education. However, important changes in the content are needed to accomodate the rapidly evolving knowledge base, the increasingly varied sites of care, and the changing patient populations. What is called for is a broader approach which will promote curriculum flexibility to meet these changing needs taking into account treatment sites, research advances, altered patient demography, and the radical change in the financing of medical care and medical education. Equally important are mechanisms to enhance curricula to meet the needs of minorities seeking to enter the profession. The increased use of secondary sources of data and of longitudinal data will require traditional clinical supervision and didiactic seminars to be expanded to include clinical pathology, internal medicine, endocrinological, neurological, sleep, and imaging components. Greater emphasis will be placed on looking at patients over time, and computers will become central in amassing such data. Increasing numbers of educational decisions will be based on evaluative research, and may lead to better undertanding of the use of role models, the relation of affect to cognition, and the intuition that makes some clinicians great. Thus, the Work Group recommended:

1. All psychiatric residents should have a required experience in planning and/or conducting empirical research.
2. All research-intensive departments of psychiatry should have a formal track for residents interested in research careers. These departments should serve as regional resources, collaborating with other departments in their area to enable qualified and interested residents to pursue these tracks.
3. Residency training programs should include training in new technologies such as computers, video, and telecommunications

to facilitate further education (through the use of literature searches and computer bulletin boards on research) and future practice (through computerized test orders, billing, etc.). The Residency Review Committee, through the Special Requirements (Essentials) for Residency Training in Psychiatry, should require residency training programs to maintain an acceptable level of computer and library resources.

4. Residency programs should have curriculum committees to monitor new developments and determine whether they warrant incorporation into curricula; residency evaluation committees should be established to evaluate faculty and teaching methods as well as trainees.
5. Residency programs should include instruction in ethnicity, transcultural issues, and the needs of unserserved populations as they relate to patient care.

PROGRAM PLANNING: CHANGING CLINICAL SETTINGS

Presenters: Anthony Reading, M.D.
Jerry M. Wiener, M.D.

Facilitator: Joseph Bloom, M.D.

Reporter: Brian B. Doyle, M.D.

While the site of practice has an effect upon what is practiced and the knowledge base that is necessary, it may not be essential or practical to expose all residents to all types of service settings. One approach to the "settings" problem is to isolate those skills which are essential to functioning in a variety of clinical systems, and ensure that residents acquire those skills during the course of the residency, although not necessarily on site. For example, skills required to practice in Health Maintenance Organizations (HMOs) may include: triage experience in psychiatric diagnosis; supervision of psychotropic medication administration by primary care physicians; supervision of staff; direct management of complex cases in acute settings; and experience in short-term individual and group psychotherapy. Residents can acquire all of these skills in current and traditional settings and successfully transpose them to the HMO.

With the foregoing as the model, the Work Group suggested:

1. Residents must be assigned a variety of clinical settings, representative of acceptable current contemporary modes. However, before such assignments are made, faculty should judge the proposed training settings primarily (but not exclusively) by how they facilitate training goals. Such experience should be well supervised by on-site psychiatrist supervisors assigned by the training director/committee.
2. There is a need for training for practice in new service settings such as HMOs, IPAs, and other nontraditional sites. Seminars on the varieties of psychiatric practice should be included in all residency training programs. Existing "transition to practice" seminars given in many programs also should address newly developing service delivery settings.
3. Proposed settings should be evaluated on multiple criteria, including whether they provide opportunities for the resident to acquire an adequate knowledge base, a clear learning task, a

nurturant environment with appropriate role models, and whether there is congruence between the tasks required in the setting and educational requirements.

PROGRAM PLANNING: ROLE OF PSYCHOTHERAPY TRAINING

Presenters: Richard Simons, M.D.
Gary Tucker, M.D.

Facilitator: Louis Faillace, M.D.

Reporter: Gordon Strauss, M.D.

There is growing pressure on residency programs to accomodate increasing amounts of information and experience into a curriculum of limited length. As the result, decisions to reduce or eliminate clinical experiences must be made. Questions have been raised about whether psychotherapy training is one of the experiences that should be curtailed. Among the issues raised regarding psychotherapy are its efficacy and whether psychotherapy skills reside primarily with psychiatrists, since many other clinicians practice psychotherapy. The group:

1. Affirmed the essential role of both longand short-term psychotherapy experiences in the training of psychiatrists for a biopsychosocial approach to treatment.
2. Agreed that residents need to be exposed to the principles, conceptual paradigms, and evidence for the efficacy and outcome of various schools of psychotherapy, including behavioral, dynamic-psychoanalytically oriented, cognitive, and hybrids such as cognitive-behavioral and interpersonal therapy.
3. Recommended that greater precision be established through the development of more efficacy data, specification of the procedures for the variety of forms of psychotherapy, criteria for competence in the conduct of psychotherapy, and evaluation procedures for resident progress toward specified competence in psychotherapy.

PROGRAM PLANNING: GENERALIST VS. SUBSPECIALIST

Presenters: Paul Fink, M.D.
Melvin Sabshin, M.D.
Joel Yager, M.D.
Patrick McKegney, M.D.

Facilitators: Normund Wong, M.D.
Theodore Nadelson, M.D.

Reporters: David Preven, M.D.
Stephen Shanfield, M.D.

Of all the issues discussed at the conference, none was the subject of more heated debate than whether the psychiatrist of the future will practice as a generalist or subspecialist. By the end of the conference, it was apparent that two different discussion groups came to entirely opposite conclusions, and that unaninimity could not be achieved. To preserve the acccuracy of the debate and the reasoning behind the disparate conclusions, the discussions and recommendations of each conference group are presented separately. Conference participants agreed that this issue will remain controversial for some time.

Discussion in Support of the Generalist Approach

For the next decade, psychiatric residency training should continue to emphasize generalist training, since this model ensures a flexible response to changing population needs, economic forces and modes of practice. Concern was voiced about premature specialization and competiton for curricular time or training funds, problems of access, and possible fragmentation of the field.

To that end, the following recommendations were made emphasizing strong general education:

1. Because the psychiatrist's central role is the diagnosis and treatment of major mental illness, residencies should continue to provide training for this role in a variety of inpatient and ambulatory care settings.
2. General psychiatrists should continue to provide the majority of treatment, although programs should have faculty with special areas of expertise to provide back-up and consultation for special problems.

3. Psychotherapy should be taught throughout the residency. All residents should be familiar with newer concepts in psychotherapeutic research.
4. Psychiatry residency training programs should provide core learning experiences in psychiatry, including experience with different age groups, a variety of service settings, specific disorders (including alcoholism and substance abuse), and a variety of areas of practice (such as consultation-liaison psychiatry, forensic psychiatry).
5. Residents should continue to receive training in understanding the relationship of the social system to mental disorders.
6. Psychiatry training programs should provide experiences in utilization and peer review.
7. Psychiatry programs should provide training in management and administration as a core experience which provides skills that are useful in a broad range of settings.
8. New teaching technologies must be created to integrate new knowledge in our field. The temptation simply to increase the content of training can fragment learning and create pedagogic chaos.
9. Considerable outcome, cost-benefit and efficacy research is needed to evaluate psychiatric treatments.

Discussion Supporting the Subspecialist Approach

The burgeoning kowledge base in psychiatry, the need to ensure that resident training includes this new information and skills, and the urgent need to assure the future quality of psychiatrists all necessitate change in the residency training process. A new model for educating the psychiatrist, encompassing both current Residency Review Committee Special Requirements (Essentials) for Residency Training in Psychiatry and the opportunity to concentrate in specialty areas, should be adopted.

The first phase should emphasize assessment and diagnosis, psychotherapy, and psychopharmacology. The evaluation of knowledge and skills in this initial phase should be based on evidence of competency established through both written exams and clinical evaluations.

In phase two, residents would pursue an area of concentration, studying with a faculty member with subspecialty expertise in that area for six months to a full year. Upon satisfactory completion of this focused work, residents would receive a certificate of concentration in that area. This experience might be followed by one or two additional years of fellowship training, upon completion of which residents would be awarded a diploma, and be eligible to participate in a rigorous certifying examination in the subspecialty.

Subspecialty designation itself should be bounded by minimum requirements. Areas so defined should be required to have: a significant knowedge base and research approach, at least one national specialty society, two or more refereed journals, special procedures or skills, and formal fellowship training. Similarly, residency training programs seeking to provide subspecialty training in a particular area should have sufficient expert faculty, appropriate clinical and didactic experiences, and good documentation that the knowledge and skills of subspecialty trainees are being evaluated effectively. It is recommended that in the course of its site visit program, the Residency Review Committee for Psychiatry carefully review the qualifications of faculty to asure that adequate subspecialty depth and breadth exist before subspecialty programs are established under the foregoing model.

FINANCING ISSUES

Presenters: Steven S. Sharfstein, M.D.
Alan Beigel, M.D.
Howard H. Goldman, M.D.
William Webb, M.D.

Facilitators: Paul Rodenhauser, M.D.
William Sledge, M.D.

Reporters: Mina Dulcan, M.D.
Robert Hales, M.D.

Psychiatric educators must engage directly in public policy decision-making concerning the funding of graduate medical education. They must adopt a proactive posture to ensure that psychiatric residency training programs are not the victims of new health care financing arrangements and service delivery systems. The goals of clinical training must be specified within the context of changing economics. To that end, Work Group recommendations regarding the future financing of graduate psychiatric education centered around increasing understanding of health care financing and its effect on psychiatry, training program content, and funding sources.

Increased Knowledge Base

1. The profession should begin to gather data to identify the precise costs and benefits of graduate medical education in psychiatry.
2. The American Psychiatric Association (APA) should develop a consultation service to training programs to address financing issues. At the same time, APA should develop data regarding existing financial arrangements between training programs and service settings and make the findings available to the field.
3. Psychiatric educators must become more knowledgeable about health care financing issues affecting their teaching facility. They must become actively involved in the fiscal affairs of the settings in which they work.

Training Program Content

1. Psychiatric educators should determine what should be taught to residents, in what setting(s) that training can best occur, and then seek funding from those settings to support the training activities.
2. Psychiatrists should be trained for flexibility and should be able to function in different settings, since patients of the future will utilize psychiatric services differently.
3. Residents should participate in new prepaid and corporate medical settings such as HMOs as well as in non-traditional health care systems and systems not affected by current reimbursement limitations.
4. Opportunities should be developed for residents and other psychiatrists to study the economic effects of various health care delivery systems.
5. Residents' awareness of economic issues should not preclude equal awareness of questions of social good when market forces may distort medical need.

Future Funding Sources for Graduate Medical Education

1. Because Medicare has been an important funding source for residency training, the profession should seek to maintain the indirect reimbursement rate for teaching hospitals under this program. Better sets of criteria under which hospitals become eligible for differential reimbursement as teaching facilities should be developed, as should better distinctions between hospital operational costs and medical education costs.
2. State or local governments should directly fund the costs of medical education in facilities treating populations for whom the government entity provides health insurance or reimbursement.
3. Teaching hospitals should be reimbursed by third-party payers at rates reflecting their educational costs.
4. Foundations, industry, and private philanthropy will play an increasingly important role in providing support to teaching hospitals, and should be encouraged actively to do so.
5. Psychiatric educators should work to ensure that the costs of financing residency training activities are shared by those individuals, public and private facilities, and others who benefit financially or otherwise from the clinical services provided by psychiatric residents.

EVALUATION: EXAMINATIONS

Presenters: Russell Gardner, Jr., M.D.
Richard I. Shader, M.D.

Facilitator: John E. Adams, M.D.

Reporter: Stephen C. Scheiber, M.D.

Examinations serve multiple purposes that should not be confused. Individual certification, for example, should not be confused with program assessment. Similarly, evaluation methodologies should be specific to particular tasks. Newer technologies should be explored and implemented as appropriate. With these goals in mind, the Work Group suggested that the current evaluative systems be redeveloped around the following recommendations:

1. In-service training examinations such as the Psychiatric Residency In-Training Examination (PRITE) should be reserved for individual and program assessment and remediation, and should not be utilized for individual pass/fail purposes. The American College of Psychiatrists should develop policies to encourage faculty access to results to facilitate remedial action.
2. The Part I written examination of the American Board of Psychiatry and Neurology should not be moved into the final year of residency training.
3. A cognitive, critical clinical incidents examination should be developed and evaluated. Successful completion of this examination should be used as a criterion for graduation from a residency program.
4. Chairmen of departments of psychiatry and residency training directors should complete annual, formal clinical skills evaluations of residents. Mechanisms to increase faculty objectivity should be developed.
5. The APA should play a leadership role in organizing an educational consortium comprised of major national psychiatric training and practice organizations to develop policies regarding evaluation of residents and criteria for promotion and graduation. Additionally, this consortium should collect or develop models of clinical assessment involving a clinical critical incidents exam.

6. Faculty should review residents' clinical experience logs for accuracy and appropriateness to assure that minimum standards are being met. Patient examples from the log could be utilized in the annual evaluation of resident clinical skills acquisition.

EVALUATION: PROGRAM ACCREDITATION REQUIREMENTS

Presenters: Arnold Cooper, M.D.
John A. Talbott, M.D.

Facilitator: Norbert B. Enzer, M.D.

Reporter: Roger Peele, M.D.

The Special Requirements (Essentials) for Residency Training in Psychiatry should be designed to ensure the quality of the academic environments in which psychiatric education occurs through regular evaluation. While it is important to describe certain core educational goals, individual programs should have substantial flexibility in curriculum design and clinical experience to encourage innovation and to capitalized on program strengths. At the same time, it is important to ensure that the residency environment is characterized by an atmosphere of inquiry and scholarship, demanding the attainment of certain standards of skills and knowledge. A program should be sensitive to individual needs of residents, and it should be supportive of personal and professional growth. Thus, the following recommendations were made by the Work Group:

1. Evaluation of psychiatric residency programs should only be undertaken by psychiatrists who are expert in psychiatric education and who have sufficient time to evaluate an individual program in depth.
2. Faculty-to-resident ratios should be established as should evidence of accessibility of the faculty to residents. Faculty should reflect a breadth and distribution of orientations, skills, and interests; faculty must be role models for ethical and professional behavior.
3. Faculty should document evidence of professional growth through scholarship, research, professional achievement, and public service.
4. Programs must isolate the skills that are essential to function in varied clinical settings and then to ensure that residents acquire those skills during the course of their residency, though not necessarily on-site.
5. Residents should be fully capable of assessing and making appropriate recommendations and referrals of psychiatric patients

in at least the following categories: children, adolescents, geriatric, chronically ill, alcohol and substance abusing patients, and medically and surgically ill patients with psychiatric problems.

6. Program evaluation should be an ongoing process including: careful documentation of residents' progress; regular evaluation of residents' knowledge, skills, and attitudes; and regular evaluation of the program components.

APPENDIX 2

THE RALEIGH CONFERENCE: PARTICIPANTS

STEERING COMMITTEE

Carol C. Nadelson, M.D.—*Chairperson*

Carolyn B. Robinowitz, M.D.

Alan Barnes, M.D.

Jonathan Borus, M.D.

Donald Fidler, M.D.

Jerald Kay, M.D.

Stefan Stein, M.D.

Allan Tasman, M.D.

PARTICIPANTS

(S = Steering Committee; P = Presenter; R = Reporter; F = Facilitator)

John E. Adams, M.D. (F)
Department of Psychiatry
University of Florida
Box J256
Gainesville, FL

Cheryl S. Al Mateen, M.D.
1219 E. Johnson Street
Philadelphia PA

James Ballenger, M.D.
Department of Psychiatry
Medical University of South Carolina
Charleston, SC

Lawrence Banta, M.D.
5110 Webster
Omaha, NE

Alan Barnes, M.D. (S)
Department of Psychiatry
University of MA Medical Center
55 Lake Avenue North
Worcester, MA

Paul Barreira, M.D.
11 Ferncroft Road
Waban, MA

Philip Bashook, Ed.D
School of Health Science
Michael Reese Hospital
Lake Shore Drive at 31st Street
Chicago, IL

Allan Beigel, M.D. (P)
30 Camino Espanol
Tucson, AZ

Irma Bland, M.D.
666 N. Lake Shore Drive
Chicago, IL

Joseph D. Bloom, M.D. (F)
Department of Psychiatry
University of Oregon Health Science Center
3181 SW Sam Jackson Park Road
Portland OR

Susan Blumenthal, M.D.
4387 Embassy Park Drive, NW
Washington, DC

Jonathan Borus, M.D. (S)
Department of Psychiatry
Massachusetts General Hospital
Fruit Street
Boston, MA

Donald B. Brown, M.D.
Morrisania Neighborhood Family Community Center
1225 Gerard Avenue
Bronx, NY

Leslie Champlin
Office of Public Affairs
American Psychiatric Association

Sara Charles, M.D.
P.O. Box 6998
Chicago, IL

Gordon Clark, M.D.
Lakes Region Health Center
Laconia NH

Richard Cohen, M.D.
WPIC
3811 O'Hara Street
Pittsburgh, PA

Arnold Cooper, M.D. (P)
Payne Whitney Psychiatric
Clinic
525 E. 68th Street
New York, NY

Miles Crowder, M.D.
Department of Psychiatry
Vanderbilt University
Nashville, TN

Leah Dickstein, M.D.
University of Louisville School
of Medicine
Bldg A, Rm. 214
Louisville, KY

Paul R. Dince, M.D.
15 West 81st Street
New York, NY

Brian Doyle, M.D. (R)
1325 18th St, NW
Washington, DC

Mina K. Dulcan, M.D. (R)
716 St. James Street
Pittsburgh PA

James Eaton, M.D.
2040 Belmont Rd., NW
Washington, DC

Joseph T. English, M.D.
Department of Psychiatry
St. Vincent's Hospital
203 West 12th Street
New York, NY

Norbert B. Enzer, M.D. (F)
College of Human Medicine
Michigan State University
East Lansing, MI

Louis Faillace, M.D. (F)
Department of Psychiatry
University of Texas Medical
School
P.O. Box 20708
Houston, TX

Larry Faulkner, M.D.
Oregon Health Science Center
3181 SW Sam Jackson Park
Road
Portland, OR

Joel Feiner, M.D.
Bronx Psychiatric Center
1500 Waters Place
Bronx, NY

Barry Fenton, M.D.
4722 Swiss Avenue
Dallas, TX

Robert C. Fernandez, M.D. (P)
11740 Lipsey Road
Tampa, FL

Donald Fidler, M.D. (S, P)
Route 5, Box 230-G
Chapel Hill, NC

Paul Fink, M.D. (P)
Philadelphia Psychiatric Center
Ford Road and Monument
Avenue
Philadelphia, PA

Janice Forster, M.D
WPIC
3811 O'Hara Street
Pittsburgh, PA

Mary Ellen Foti, M.D.
12 Pond Lane, #41
Arlington, MA

Marc Frader, M.D.
26 Norfolk Road
Arlington, MA

Richard Frances, M.D.
21 Bloomingdale Road
White Plains, NY

Shervert H. Frazier, M.D. (P)
McLean Hospital
115 Mill Street
Belmont, MA

Robert Friedel, M.D.
Charter Medical Corporation
1500 Westbrook Avenue
Richmond, VA

Linda Ganzini, M.D.
8225 Southwest 39th Street
Portland, OR

Russell Gardner, Jr., M.D. (P)
Department of Psychiatry and
Behavioral Science
University of Texas Medical
Branch
Galveston, TX

George Ginsberg, M.D.
4 East 89th Street
New York, NY

Marcia K. Goin, M.D.
1245 Wilshire Boulevard
Los Angeles, CA

David Goldberg, M.D.
Department of Psychiatry
University of Connecticut
Health Science Center
Farmington, CT

Howard H. Goldman, M.D. (P)
10600 Trotters Trail
Potomac, MD

Jean Goodwin, M.D.
4105 N. Lake Drive
Shorewood, WI

Robert Grillo, Jr., M.D.
7 Arapahoe Road
W. Hartford, CT

Frederick Guggenheim, M.D.
4301 West Markham
Little Rock, AR

Melvyn Haas, M.D.
NIMH, Room 7C10
5600 Fishers Lane
Rockville, MD

Robert Hales, M.D. (R)
Department of Psychiatry
USUHS
4301 Jones Bridge Road
Bethesda, MD

James Halikas, M.D.
University of Minnesota
Hospitals and Clinics
P.O. Box 393
Minneapolis, MN

Seymour Halleck, M.D.
Department of Psychiatry
University of North Carolina
Chapel Hill, NC

Donald Hammersley, M.D.
Deputy Medical Director
American Psychiatric
Association

Alma Herndon
Psychiatric News
American Psychiatric
Association

Peter Henderson, M.D.
WPIC
3811 O'Hara Street
Pittsburgh, PA

James R. Hilliard M.D. (R)
Department of Psychiatry
University of Cincinnati
231 Bethesda Avenue
Cincinnati, OH

Jeffrey Houpt, M.D. (F)
Georgia Mental Health
Institution
1256 Briarcliff Road, NE
Atlanta, GA

David Janowsky, M.D.
Department of Psychiatry
UCSD
La Jolla, CA

David Joseph, M.D.
1094 R Street NW
Washington, DC

Edward Joseph, M.D.
Mt. Sinai School of Medicine
Department of Psychiatry
1 East 100th Street
New York, NY

David Katz, M.D.
McLean Hospital
115 Mill St Belmont, MA

Steven Katz, M.D.
Office of Mental Health
44 Holland Avenue
Albany, NY

Edward Kaufman, M.D.
Department of Psychiatry
Building 53
101 City Drive South
Orange, CA

Jerald Kay, M.D. (S)
University of Cincinnati
Department of Psychiatry
231 Bethesda Avenue
Cincinnati, OH

Rena Kay, M.D.
419 Rose Hill Avenue
Cincinnati, OH

Howard Kibel, M.D.
NY Hospital-Cornell Medical
Center
Westchester Division
21 Bloomingdale Road
White Plains, NY

Chase P. Kimball, M.D.
Department of Psychiatry
University of Chicago
950 E. 59th Street
Chicago, IL

Gerald Klerman, M.D.
525 East 68th Street
New York, NY

James Krajeski, M.D.
2001 Union Street
San Francisco, CA

Donald Langsley, M.D. (P)
ABMS, Suite 805
One American Plaza
Evanston, IL

Richard Lanman, M.D.
275 Hospital Parkway
Suite 375
San Jose, CA

Aaron Lazare, M.D.
95 Dorset Road
Waban, MA

Robert Leon, M.D.
Department of Psychiatry
University Texas Health
Sciences Center
7703 Floyd Curl Drive
San Antonio, TX

Norman B. Levy, M.D.
Liaison Psychiatric Division
Westchester County Medical
Center
Valhalla, NY

Don Lipsett, M D.
156 Griggs Road
Brookline, MA

Benjamin Liptzin, M.D.
McLean Hospital
115 Mill Street
Belmont, MA

James Lomax, M.D.
Department of Psychiatry
Baylor College of Medicine
One Baylor Plaza
Houston, TX

Earl Loschen, M.D.
Department of Psychiatry
SIU School of Medicine
P.O. Box 3926
Springfield, IL

James Lurie, M.D.
1417 E. Aloha
Seattle, WA

Philip Margolis, M.D.
228 Riverview Drive
Ann Arbor, MI

John Markowitz, M.D.
Payne Whitney Clinic
525 East 68th Street
New York, NY

James Mathis, M.D.
Department of Psychiatric
Medicine
East Carolina University
Medical School
Greenville, NC

Christine McGuire
8 South Michigan Avenue
Chicago, IL

F. Patrick McKegney, M.D. (P)
Montefiore Medical Center
111 East 210th Street
Bronx, NY

Robert F. Meyer, M.D.
5040 North 15th Avenue #305
Phoenix, AZ

Roger Meyer, M.D.
15 Uplands Drive
West Hartford, CT

Robert A. Moore, M.D.
Vista Hill Foundation
3420 Camino Del Rio N. #100
San Diego, CA

Emily Mumford, Ph.D.
NY State Psychiatric Institute
New School for Social Research
65 Fifth Avenue
New York, NY

Michael Myers, M.D.
Department of Psychiatry
Shaughnessy Hospital
4500 Oak Street
Vancouver, Canada

Carol C. Nadelson, M.D. (S)
Department of Psychiatry
Tufts University School of Medicine
250 Washington Street
Boston, MA

Theodore Nadelson, M.D. (F)
Boston VA Medical Center
150 S. Huntington Avenue
Boston, MA

Robert Niven, M.D.
Comprehensive Psychiatric Services, Inc.
21415 Civic Center Drive
Suite 119
Southfield, MI

Malkah T. Notman, M.D.
54 Clark Road
Brookline, MA

Roger Peele, M.D. (R)
12919 Asbury Drive
Ft. Washington, MD

Irving Phillips, M.D.
Department of Psychiatry
University of California Medical Center
San Francisco, CA

Robert T. M. Phillips, M.D.
366 Central Avenue
New Haven, CT

Harold Alan Pincus, M.D.
Deputy Medical Director
Office of Research
American Psychiatric Association

David Preven, M.D. (R)
40 Iselin Terrace
Larchmont, NY

Ray Purkis
Director, Advertising Sales
American Psychiatric Association

H. Paul Putman, M.D.
1188 Village Creek Lane #4
Mount Pleasant, SC

Frank T. Rafferty, M.D.
VP for Medical Affairs
Healthcare International
P.O. Box 4008
Austin, TX

Anthony Reading, M.D. (P)
Department of Psychiatry
University of S. Florida
1201 N. 30th Street
Tampa, FL

Ronald Rieder, M.D.
NY State Psychiatric Institute
177 West 168th Street
New York, NY

Carolyn B. Robinowitz, M.D. (S)
Deputy Medical Director
Office of Education
American Psychiatric Association

Luther Robinson, M.D.
Howard University Hospital
2041 Georgia Avenue, NW
Washington, DC

Paul Rodenhauser, M.D. (F)
1211 Fair Hills Avenue
Suite 315
Dayton, OH

Melvin Sabshin, M.D. (P)
Medical Director
American Psychiatric Association

Jose Santiago, M.D.
5112 N. Via Condesa
Tucson, AZ

Alberto Santos, M.D.
Department of Psychiatry
Medical University of South Carolina
171 Ashley Avenue
Charleston, SC

Stephen Scheiber, M.D. (R)
ABPN, Suite 808
One American Plaza
Evanston, IL

Donald Scherl, M.D.
450 Clarkson Avenue
Box 1
Brooklyn, NY

Randolph Schiffer, M.D.
University of Rochester Medical Center
300 Crittenden Boulevard
Rochester, NY

Peter Silberfarb, M.D.
Dartmouth-Hitchcock Medical Center
Hanover, NH

Richard Simons, M.D. (P)
38 Martin Lane
Englewood CO

William Sledge, M.D. (F)
Yale University School of Medicine
34 Park Street
New Haven, CT

Selwyn M. Smith, M.D.
Department of Psychiatry
Royal Ottawa Hospital
1145 Carling Avenue
Ottawa, Canada

Jeanne Spurlock, M.D.
Deputy Medical Director
Office of Minority and National Affairs
American Psychiatric Association

Stefan Stein, M.D. (S)
Department of Psychiatry
NY Hospital-Cornell Medical Center
Westchester Division
21 Bloomingdale Road
White Plains, NY

Terry Stein, M.D.
Department of Psychiatry
Michigan Street University
East Fee Hall
East Lansing, MI

Lawrence A. Stone, M.D.
4606 Centerview Drive
Suite 266
Sabine Building
San Antonio, TX

John Schowalter, M.D.
Yale Child Study Center
New Haven, CT

Ann Seiden, M.D.
Department of Psychiatry
Cook County Hospital
1835 W. Harrison, B Building
Chicago, IL

Richard Shader, M.D. (P)
Department of Psychiatry
Tufts University School of Medicine
Box 1007
Boston, MA

Mohammad Shafii, M.D.
6305 Shadowood Court
Prospect, KY

Charles Shamoian, M.D.
NY Hospital-Cornell Medical Center
Westchester Division
21 Bloomingdale Road
White Plains, NY

Stephan Shanfield, M.D. (R)
Department of Psychiatry
University of TX Health Science Center
7703 Floyd Curl Drive
San Antonio, TX

Steven S. Sharfstein, M.D. (P)
Sheppard and Enoch Pratt Hospital
6501 N. Charles Street
Baltimore, MD

Kailie Shaw, M.D. (P)
4145 Northmeadow Circle
Tampa, FL

Gordon Strauss, M.D. (R)
4929 Gloria Avenue
Encino, CA

Zebulon Taintor, M.D. (P)
19 East 93rd Street
New York, NY

John A. Talbott, M.D. (P)
200 Goodwood Gardens
Baltimore, MD

Allan Tasman, M.D. (S)
University of Connecticut Health Center
Department of Psychiatry
Farmington, CT

Kenneth Tardiff, M.D.
Cornell University Medical College
1300 York Avenue
New York, NY

Bryce Templeton, M.D.
Jefferson Medical College
1015 Walnut Street
3d Floor, Curtis Building
Philadelphia, PA

James W. Thompson, Ph.D.
NIMH, Room 18C-22
5600 Fishers Lane
Rockville, MD

Patti Tighe, M.D.
2800 N. Lake Shore Drive
Chicago, IL

Gary Tucker, M.D. (P)
Department of Psychiatry and Behavioral Science
University of Washington
RP10-10
Seattle, WA

Paul Wachter, M.D.
725 Chester Way
Hillsborough CA

Preston Walker, M.D.
5207 Hawksbury Lane
Raleigh, NC

William Webb, M.D. (P)
Institute of Living
200 Retreat Avenue
Hartford, CT

Sidney H. Weissman, M.D.
Department of Psychiatry
Michael Reese Hospital
Lake Shore Drive at 31st Street
Chicago, IL

Ronald Weller, M.D.
Department of Psychiatry
Ohio State University Hospital
473 West 12th Avenue
Columbus, OH

Elizabeth Weller, M.D.
Department of Psychiatry
Ohio State University Hospital
473 West 12th Avenue
Columbus, OH

Jerry Wiener, M.D. (P)
Department of Psychiatry and Behavioral Science
George Washington University
2130 Pennsylvania Avenue, NW
Washington, DC

Albert Williams, M.D., Ph.D.
Rand Corporation
1708 Main Street
Santa Monica, CA

Donald H. Williams, M.D.
Room A223, East Fee Hall
Michigan State University
East Lansing, MI

Daniel Winstead, M.D.
Department of Psychiatry
Tulane University Medical Center
1430 Tulane Avenue
New Orleans, LA

Normund Wong, M.D. (F)
Letterman Army Medical Center
San Francisco, CA

Harry Wright, M.D.
William S. Hall Psychiatric Institute
P.O. Box 202
Columbia, SC

Joel Yager, M.D. (P)
UCLA-NPI
760 Westwood Plaza
Los Angeles, CA

Leonard Zegans, M.D.
Langley Porter Institute
401 Parnassus Avenue
San Francisco, CA

Veva Zimmerman, M.D.
12 East 87th Street, Suite 2B
New York, NY